theclinics.com

ULTRASOUND CLINICS

Breast Ultrasound

Guest Editor
GARY J. WHITMAN, MD

October 2006 • Volume 1 • Number 4

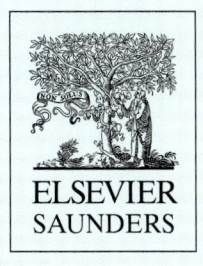

ELSEVIER
SAUNDERS

An imprint of Elsevier, Inc
PHILADELPHIA LONDON TORONTO MONTREAL SYDNEY TOKYO

W.B. SAUNDERS COMPANY
A Division of Elsevier Inc.

1600 John F. Kennedy Boulevard • Suite 1800 • Philadelphia, Pennsylvania 19103-2899

http://www.theclinics.com

ULTRASOUND CLINICS Volume 1, Number 4
October 2006 ISSN 1556-858X, ISBN 1-4160-3937-6

Editor: Barton Dudlick

Copyright © 2007 Elsevier Inc. All rights reserved. No part of this publication may be reproduced or transmitted in any form or by any means, electronic or mechanical, including photocopy, recording, or any information retrieval system, without written permission from the publisher.

Single photocopies of single articles may be made for personal use as allowed by national copyright laws. Permission of the publisher and payment of a fee is required for all other photocopying, including multiple or systematic copying, copying for advertising or promotional purposes, resale, and all forms of document delivery. Special rates are available for educational institutions that wish to make photocopies for non-profit educational classroom use. Permissions may be sought directly from Elsevier's Rights Department in Philadelphia, PA, USA at Tel.: (+1) 215-239-3804;, Fax: (+1) 215-239-3805; E-mail: healthpermissions@elsevier.com. Requests may also be completed on-line via the Elsevier homepage (http://www.elsevier.com/locate/permissions). In the USA, users may clear permissions and make payments through the Copyright Clearance Center, Inc., 222 Rosewood Drive, Danvers, MA 01923, USA; Tel.: (+1) 978-750-8400; Fax: (+1) 978-750-4744, and in the UK through the Copyright Licensing Agency Rapid Clearance Service (CLARCS), 90 Tottenham Court Road, London W1P 0LP, UK; Tel.: (+44) 171-436-5931; Fax: (+44) 171-436-3986. Others countries may have a local reprographic rights agency for payments.

Reprints: For copies of 100 or more, of articles in this publication, please contact the Commercial Reprints Department, Elsevier Inc., 360 Park Avenue South, New York, New York 10010-1710. Tel.: (+1) 212-633-3813; Fax: (+1) 212-462-1935 Email: reprints@elsevier.com

The ideas and opinions expressed in *Ultrasound Clinics* do not necessarily reflect those of the Publisher. The Publisher does not assume any responsibility for any injury and/or damage to persons or property arising out of or related to any use of the material contained in this periodical. The reader is advised to check the appropriate medical literature and the product information currently provided by the manufacturer of each drug to be administered to verify the dosage, the method and duration of administration, or contraindications. It is the responsibility of the treating physician or other health care professional, relying on independent experience and knowledge of the patient, to determine drug dosages and the best treatment for the patient. Mention of any product in this issue should not be construed as endorsement by the contributors, editors, or the Publisher of the product or manufacturers' claims.

Ultrasound Clinics (ISSN 1556-858X) is published quarterly by W.B. Saunders, 360 Park Avenue South, New York, NY 10010-1710. Months of publication are January, April, July, and October. Business and editorial offices: 1600 John F. Kennedy Boulevard, Suite 1800, Philadelphia, Pennsylvania 19103-2899. Accounting and circulation offices: 6277 Sea Harbor Drive, Orlando, FL 32887-4800. Periodicals postage paid at New York NY, and additional mailing offices. Subscription prices are USD 162 per year for US individuals, USD 223 per year for US institutions, USD 81 per year for US students and residents, USD 184 per year for Canadian individuals, USD 212 per year for Canadian institutions, USD 184 per year for international individuals, USD 244 per year for international institutions, and USD 92 per year for Canadian and foreign students/residents. To receive student/resident rate, orders must be accompanied by name of affiliated institution, date of term, and the signature of program/residency coordinator on institution letterhead. Orders will be billed at individual rate until proof of status is received. Foreign air speed delivery is included in all Clinics subscription prices. All prices are subject to change without notice. **POSTMASTER:** Send address changes to *Ultrasound Clinics,* Elsevier Periodicals Customer Service, 6277 Sea Harbor Drive, Orlando, FL 32887-4800. **Customer Service: 1-800-654-2452 (US).** From outside of the US, call (+1) 407-345-4000.

Printed in the United States of America.

BREAST ULTRASOUND

EDITORIAL BOARD

VIKRAM S. DOGRA, MD
Professor of Radiology and Associate Chair of Education and Research; Department of Imaging Sciences; Director, Division of Ultrasound, and Department of Radiology, University of Rochester School of Medicine and Dentistry, Rochester, New York

DEBORAH LEVINE, MD
Associate Professor, Department of Radiology, Harvard Medical School; Associate Radiologist-in-Chief of Academic Affairs, Beth Israel Deaconess Medical Center, Boston, Massachusetts

GUEST EDITOR

GARY J. WHITMAN, MD
Associate Professor, Department of Radiology, The University of Texas M. D. Anderson Cancer Center, Houston, Texas

CONTRIBUTORS

WENDIE A. BERG, MD, PhD, FACR
Breast Imaging Consultant, American Radiology Services, Johns Hopkins Green Spring, Lutherville, Maryland

ANGELICA CANTU
Undergraduate Student, Texas A&M University, College Station, Texas

GILDA CARDENOSA, MD
Professor, Department of Radiology, Virginia Commonwealth University, Richmond, Virginia; Director of Breast Imaging, Department of Radiology, Medical College of Virginia Hospital, Richmond, Virginia

BASAK ERGUVAN-DOGAN, MD
Fellow, Department of Diagnostic Radiology, The University of Texas M. D. Anderson Cancer Center, Houston, Texas

BEVERLY E. HASHIMOTO, MD, FACR
Section Head, Ultrasound, Virginia Mason Medical Center, Seattle, Washington

PHAN T. HUYNH, MD
Medical Director, Women's Center, St. Luke's Episcopal Hospital, Houston, Texas

SAVITRI KRISHNAMURTHY, MD
Associate Professor, Department of Pathology, Department of Pathology, The University of Texas M. D. Anderson Cancer Center, Houston, Texas

PARUL PATEL, MS
Medical Student, State University of New York Upstate Medical University, Syracuse, New York

GARY J. WHITMAN, MD
Associate Professor, Department of Radiology, Department of Diagnostic Radiology, The University of Texas M. D. Anderson Cancer Center, Houston, Texas

JOELLA WILSON, BS
Medical Student, The University of Kansas School of Medicine, Kansas City, Kansas

B. SYBILLE WOEL, MD
Washington Radiology Associates, Washington, District of Columbia

WEI TSE YANG, MBBS, FRCR
Associate Professor, Department of Radiology, Department of Diagnostic Radiology, The University of Texas M. D. Anderson Cancer Center, Houston, Texas

BREAST ULTRASOUND

Contents

Preface
Gary J. Whitman

xi

Mammographic–Sonographic Correlation
Wendie A. Berg and B. Sybille Woel

567

> Accurate correlation of mammographic and sonographic findings first requires complete diagnostic mammographic work-up and development of an appropriate differential diagnosis before sonographic evaluation. The finding of interest should be characterized as a mass, asymmetry, architectural distortion, suspicious calcifications, or a combination of these features. Mammographic and sonographic location, size, shape, and margins should be concordant and carefully correlated to avoid errors. Unique issues arise in women who have nipple discharge, implants, and palpable masses. This article examines each of these issues in detail.

Breast Ultrasound MR Imaging Correlation
Basak Erguvan-Dogan and Gary J. Whitman

593

> Sonography and ultrasound-guided biopsy should be performed for suspicious breast lesions identified on MR imaging before performing MR imaging–guided breast biopsy. This article reviews the literature to date on the use of targeted sonography for identification of MR imaging–detected breast lesions. A flow chart is provided depicting suggested management of breast lesions with suspicious enhancement detected by MR imaging alone.

Ultrasound-Guided Breast Biopsies
Gary J. Whitman, Basak Erguvan-Dogan, Wei Tse Yang, Joella Wilson, Parul Patel, and Savitri Krishnamurthy

603

> Currently, nearly all breast biopsies are performed with percutaneous techniques, and nearly all biopsies of masses are ultrasound guided. This article reviews ultrasound-guided breast biopsies. Ultrasound-guided core biopsies, vacuum-assisted biopsies, and fine-needle aspirations are discussed along with ultrasound-guided marker placement and imaging–pathologic correlation. The advantages and disadvantages of ultrasound-guided biopsies are covered, along with preprocedural preparations.

Cysts, Cystic Lesions, and Papillary Lesions 617
Gilda Cardenosa

This article discusses the imaging appearance and appropriate treatment of simple cysts; complex cystic masses; oil cysts; other fluid collections, including postoperative and collections, galactoceles, and abscesses; solitary papillomas and multiple peripheral papillomas; and papillary carcinoma.

Sonography of Ductal Carcinoma in Situ 631
Beverly E. Hashimoto

One of the most commonly identified malignancies, ductal carcinoma in situ (DCIS), generally is discovered on screening mammography in the form of clustered microcalcifications. Today, using higher frequencies and advanced contrast techniques, sonologists can provide additional imaging information beyond that obtained with mammography. Sonography may reveal DCIS masses that are mammographically occult. Sonography may reveal other DCIS features such as calcifications, abnormal ducts, masses associated with fluid collections, and multicystic masses. Sonographically guided interventional procedures are faster and easier for patients to tolerate than procedures performed using mammography or MR imaging guidance and may improve the patient's diagnostic experience.

Sonography of Invasive Lobular Carcinoma 645
Gary J. Whitman, Phan T. Huynh, Parul Patel, Joella Wilson, Angelica Cantu, and Savitri Krishnamurthy

Invasive lobular carcinoma (ILC) accounts for 5% to 14% of all breast cancers. ILC may be difficult to detect on clinical examination and mammography. This article reviews the pathologic, clinical, mammographic, and MR imaging features of ILC, with an emphasis on sonography of ILC. The role of ultrasound in evaluating multicentric, multifocal, and bilateral ILC is covered, along with sonographic staging of the axillary lymph nodes.

Sonography of Unusual Breast Neoplasms 661
Wei Tse Yang

This article reviews the sonographic features of uncommon breast neoplasms and systemic conditions. Unusual nonmammary malignant tumors of the breast include primary and secondary lymphoreticular malignancies, primary and secondary sarcomas, and hematogenous metastases. Uncommon benign tumors that occur in the breast include fibromatosis, granular cell tumors, hamartomas, tubular adenomas, lactating adenomas, and pseudoangiomatous stromal hyperplasia. Some examples of non-neoplastic systemic diseases that may involve the breast include collagen vascular disease (rheumatoid arthritis, systemic lupus erythematosus, scleroderma, psoriatic arthritis, and dermatomyositis), granulomatous disease (tuberculosis and sarcoidosis), AIDS, infectious mononucleosis, diabetic fibrous mastopathy, hyperparathyroidism, and vasculitis (Wegener's granulomatosis).

Index 673

FORTHCOMING ISSUES

January 2007
Genitourinary Ultrasound
Vikram S. Dogra, MD, *Guest Editor*

April 2007
Abdominal Ultrasound
Lesile Scoutt, MD, *Guest Editor*

RECENT ISSUES

July 2006
Pediatric Ultrasound
Brian Coley, MD, *Guest Editor*

Intraoperative Ultrasonography of the Abdomen
Jonathan Kruskal, MD, and Robert Kane, MD, *Guest Editors*

April 2006
Obstetric Ultrasound
Deborah Levine, MD, *Guest Editor*

Gynecologic Ultrasound
Ruth B. Goldstein, MD, *Guest Editor*

THE CLINICS ARE NOW AVAILABLE ONLINE!

Access your subscription at:
www.theclinics.com

GOAL STATEMENT

The goal of the *Ultrasound Clinics* is to keep practicing radiologists and radiology residents up to date with current clinical practice in ultrasound by providing timely articles reviewing the state of the art in patient care.

ACCREDITATION

The *Ultrasound Clinics* is planned and implemented in accordance with the Essential Areas and Policies of the Accreditation Council for Continuing Medical Education (ACCME) through the joint sponsorship of the University of Virginia School of Medicine and Elsevier. The University of Virginia School of Medicine is accredited by the ACCME to provide continuing medical education for physicians.

The University of Virginia School of Medicine designates this educational activity for a maximum of 15 *AMA PRA Category 1 Credits*™. Physicians should only claim credit commensurate with the extent of their participation in the activity.

The American Medical Association has determined that physicians not licensed in the US who participate in this CME activity are eligible for 15 *AMA PRA Category 1 Credits*™.

Credit can be earned by reading the text material, taking the CME examination online at http://www.theclinics.com/home/cme, and completing the evaluation. After taking the test, you will be required to review any and all incorrect answers. Following completion of the test and evaluation, your credit will be awarded and you may print your certificate.

FACULTY DISCLOSURE/CONFLICT OF INTEREST

The University of Virginia School of Medicine, as an ACCME accredited provider, endorses and strives to comply with the Accreditation Council for Continuing Medical Education (ACCME) Standards of Commercial Support, Commonwealth of Virginia statutes, University of Virginia policies and procedures, and associated federal and private regulations and guidelines on the need for disclosure and monitoring of proprietary and financial interests that may affect the scientific integrity and balance of content delivered in continuing medical education activities under our auspices.

The University of Virginia School of Medicine requires that all CME activities accredited through this institution be developed independently and be scientifically rigorous, balanced and objective in the presentation/discussion of its content, theories and practices.

All authors/editors participating in an accredited CME activity are expected to disclose to the readers relevant financial relationships with commercial entities occurring within the past 12 months (such as grants or research support, employee, consultant, stock holder, member of speakers bureau, etc.). The University of Virginia School of Medicine will employ appropriate mechanisms to resolve potential conflicts of interest to maintain the standards of fair and balanced education to the reader. Questions about specific strategies can be directed to the Office of Continuing Medical Education, University of Virginia School of Medicine, Charlottesville, Virginia.

The authors/editors listed below have identified no professional or financial affiliations for themselves or their spouse/partner:
Wendie Berg, MD; Angelica Cantu; Gilda Cardenosa, MD; Basak Dogan, MD; Barton Dudlick (Acquisitions Editor); Phan Huynh, MD; Savitri Krishnamurthy, MD; Parul Patel, MD; Gary Whitman, MD (Guest Editor); Joella Wilson, MD; B. Sybille Woel, MD; and, Wei Tse Yang, MD.

The authors/editors listed below have identified the following professional or financial affiliations for themselves or their spouse/partner:
Beverly Hashimoto, MD, FACR is a consultant for Advanced Imaging Technologies; is on the advisory board for Siemens; and is a principal investigator for Phillips and DOBI in the area of breast imaging.

Disclosure of Discussion of non-FDA approved uses for pharmaceutical products and/or medical devices:
The University of Virginia School of Medicine, as an ACCME provider, requires that all faculty presenters identify and disclose any "off label" uses for pharmaceutical and medical device products. The University of Virginia School of Medicine recommends that each physician fully review all the available data on new products or procedures prior to instituting them with patients.

TO ENROLL

To enroll in the Ultrasound Clinics Continuing Medical Education program, call customer service at 1-800-654-2452 or visit us online at www.theclinics.com/home/cme. The CME program is available to subscribers for an additional fee of $205.00.

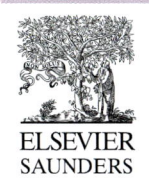

Preface

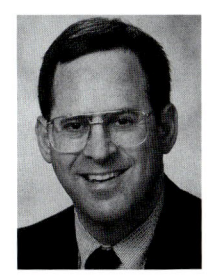

Gary J. Whitman, MD
Department of Diagnostic Radiology
The University of Texas M. D. Anderson Cancer Center
P.O. Box 301439, Unit 1350
Houston, TX 77230, USA

E-mail address:
gwhitman@di.mdacc.tmc.edu

Gary J. Whitman, MD
Guest Editor

Breast sonography is indispensable. Most breast lesions, other than small clusters of calcifications, can and may be evaluated with ultrasound. In the last decade and a half, we have witnessed tremendous progress in breast ultrasound. The days of using breast ultrasound solely to differentiate cysts from solid masses are gone forever. Breast sonography is commonly used to evaluate mammographic and palpable abnormalities, and ultrasound is often used to evaluate findings initially noted on magnetic resonance imaging (MRI). Sonography also plays a role in screening for breast cancer and in evaluating the extent of disease in the breast and the regional lymph nodes.

Nearly all breast masses are sampled with ultrasound-guided biopsy. Core biopsies, vacuum-assisted biopsies, and fine-needle aspirations are commonly performed with sonographic guidance, often followed by ultrasound-guided marker placement. In addition, sonography can be used to help guide catheters to drain abscesses or deliver radiation therapy. In some centers, ultrasound is guiding cryoablation and radiofrequency ablation of breast lesions.

Breast ultrasound can be performed just about anywhere. Although most ultrasound machines are housed in sonography rooms, breast ultrasound can be and has been performed in mammography rooms, operating rooms, surgical holding areas, emergency rooms, examination rooms, patient hospital rooms, and intensive care units. Breast ultrasound plays a major role in the daily management of women with breast diseases.

In this issue of *Ultrasound Clinics*, we explore some of the common uses of breast sonography. Drs. Berg and Woel cover mammographic-sonographic correlation in a comprehensive manner, and Dr. Dogan and I provide an update on MRI-sonographic correlation. Dr. Dogan, Dr. Yang, Joella Wilson, Parul Patel, and Dr. Krishnamurthy assisted me on an article on ultrasound-guided biopsies. Dr. Cardenosa covers cysts, cystic lesions, and papillary lesions with a practical approach, and Dr. Hashimoto provides an update on sonography of ductal carcinoma in situ. Dr. Huynh, Parul Patel, Joella Wilson, Angelica Cantu, and Dr. Krishnamurthy assisted me on an article on sonography of invasive lobular carcinoma. Finally, Dr. Yang covers sonography of unusual breast neoplasms. All of the authors did a great job, and I thank them for taking time away from other pursuits to work on *Ultrasound Clinics*. Many thanks!

Stephanie Deming and Ann Sutton in Scientific Publications at The University of Texas M. D. Anderson Cancer Center did an outstanding job editing many of the manuscripts. Barton Dudlick and his colleagues at Elsevier did a wonderful job coordinating this project, and I thank Barton for his patience. Barbara Almarez Mahinda, my administrative assistant, did an incredible job (as usual) on this project. She is indispensable! Many thanks to my wife, Susan, and my son, Sam, for their understanding and patience when Daddy was working on "the chapters." Thank you!

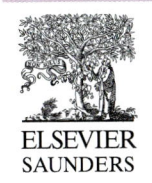

ULTRASOUND
CLINICS

Mammographic–Sonographic Correlation

Wendie A. Berg, MD, PhD[a],*, B. Sybille Woel, MD[b]

- Location
- Use of intrinsic landmarks
- Size
- Masses
- Asymmetries and architectural distortion
- Calcifications
- Inflammatory carcinoma
- Implants
- Nipple discharge
- Palpable abnormalities
- Confirming concordance
- Summary
- References

Accurate correlation of mammographic and sonographic findings first requires complete diagnostic mammographic work-up and development of an appropriate differential diagnosis before sonographic evaluation. The finding of interest should be characterized as a mass, asymmetry, architectural distortion, suspicious calcifications, or a combination of these features [1]. Mammographic and sonographic location, size, shape, and margins should be concordant and carefully correlated to avoid errors. Unique issues arise in women who have nipple discharge, implants, and palpable masses. This article examines each of these issues in detail.

Location

A key to correlating mammographic and sonographic or MR imaging findings is visualizing where a lesion should be within the breast in three dimensions and translating that visualization to the imaging modality of interest. Mammography usually is performed with the patient standing or sitting upright. Breast ultrasound usually is performed with the patient supine for the inner breast and in the contralateral decubitus position for the outer breast. MR imaging is performed with the patient prone and the breasts dependent within the coil. There are few fixed landmarks in the breast other than the nipple and chest wall: these will be used as referents.

Location of a finding on mammography is usually described by quadrant (upper outer, upper inner, lower outer, lower inner), subareolar, central, or axillary tail positions [1]. Description of location on ultrasound is usually by clock face (Fig. 1), as if a clock has been placed on the breast with 12:00 cephalad and 6:00 caudad. Thinking in terms of expected clock-face location is helpful when reviewing mammograms (Fig. 2) and facilitates successfully targeting ultrasound to mammographic abnormalities.

Triangulation is an important part of understanding the final three-dimensional clock-face location of a mammographic abnormality [2]. The mediolateral oblique (MLO) mammogram is taken at variable angles to be parallel to the individual patient's pectoral muscle, whereas for ultrasound one needs

---

[a] American Radiology Services, Johns Hopkins Green Spring, 10755 Falls Road, Suite 440, Baltimore, MD 21093, USA
[b] Washington Radiology Associates, P.C. 3015 Williams Drive, Suite 200, Fairfax, VA 22031, USA
* Corresponding author.
E-mail address: wendieberg@hotmail.com (W.A. Berg).

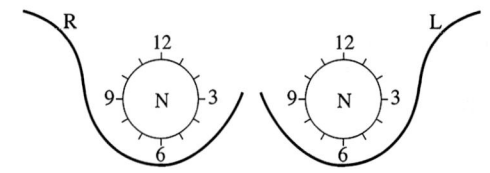

Fig. 1. Diagram shows clock-face locations by breast as used to annotate ultrasound images. (Courtesy of Wendie A. Berg, MD, PhD, FACR, Baltimore, MD. © Copyright 2006.)

to know the expected location of a lesion on a true lateral (90°) view. By triangulation, one can infer from any combination of two mammographic views (typically the craniocaudal [CC] and MLO views) where the lesion would be on the third, 90° true lateral (either mediolateral or laterome-dial) view and therefore in three dimensions within the breast (Fig. 3). Triangulation also is used to help locate a lesion in three dimensions when it is seen on only one of the routine mammographic views (ie, either the CC or the MLO view) [3]. A true lateral view is then obtained. If the lesion can be seen on both true lateral and MLO views, its position on the CC view can be inferred (see Fig. 3). Lateral lesions move lower (inferiorly) from CC to MLO to true lateral views (when viewing the true lateral image to the right of the MLO view), and medial lesions move superiorly from CC to MLO to true lateral views. (A mnemonic is "Lead falls and muffins rise.") (J.E. Meyer, MD, personal communication, 1998).

Rolled CC views can help locate a lesion seen only on the CC view [4]. In this maneuver, the top half of the breast is rolled laterally (CCRL view) or medially (CCRM view); a lesion moving with the top half of the breast is known to be in the upper breast (Fig. 4). Lesions seen only in the upper posterior breast on the MLO view are most commonly in the axillary tail region and can usually be seen on a laterally exaggerated CC view (Fig. 5).

Once the expected clock-face location is known from mammography, the distance from the nipple and the depth of the lesion from the skin must be considered. On mammography, this information usually is expressed by dividing the anteroposterior thickness of the breast into thirds (anterior, middle, or posterior depth) or as a single measurement (ie, distance from the nipple). Rather than a single mammographic measurement of depth from the nipple, to correlate better with ultrasound, it is preferable to consider the depth of the lesion (superficial, middle depth, or posterior, that is, at chest wall) relative to the skin, which may or may not correlate with depth from the nipple on mammography. For example, a lesion near the skin of the far lateral breast near the chest wall would be superficial on ultrasound but project at a posterior depth on mammography (Fig. 6). Adequate sonographic characterization of superficial lesions is facilitated by use of a glob of gel or a standoff pad so that the lesion is at least 5 to 7 mm away from the face of the transducer; even with current 12- to 15-MHz linear array transducers, the beam cannot be optimally focused more anteriorly.

Anterior lesions on mammography should be within the anterior third of the tissue on ultrasound, closer to the skin surface than the chest wall (Fig. 7). Similarly, posterior lesions close to the chest wall (but not the skin) on both mammographic views should be close to the pectoral muscle on ultrasound (Fig. 8). It also is useful to consider the distance medial or lateral and superior or inferior to the nipple on mammography to help direct targeted ultrasound (see Fig. 6). On ultrasound, the distance along the skin surface from the center of the lesion to the nipple in centimeters should be specified on the ultrasound images; the 38- or 50-mm footprint of the transducer itself can be used as a guide for reliably estimating and recording this measurement [5].

Location and distance from the nipple on ultrasound generally correlates well with

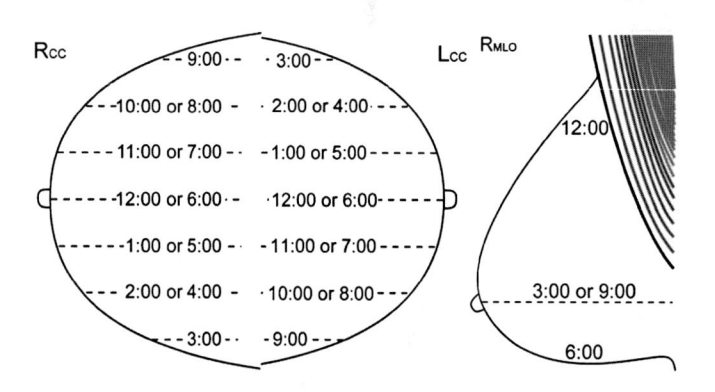

Fig. 2. Clock-face location is first inferred from the CC position of a finding, with the MLO view used predominantly to determine whether a mass is in the upper (above the nipple) or lower (below the nipple) breast. (Courtesy of Wendie A. Berg, MD, PhD, FACR, Baltimore, MD. © Copyright 2006.)

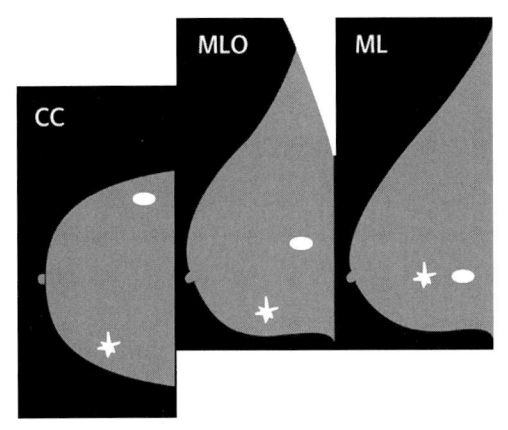

Fig. 3. Triangulation. With the nipple aligned across views and the MLO view in the center, the location of a mass visible in only two of the three mammographic projections can be inferred by triangulation. Lateral masses (eg, the oval mass in this example) will move inferiorly from CC to MLO to mediolateral views, whereas medial masses (eg, the spiculated mass in this example) will project more superiorly from CC to MLO to mediolateral views. (Courtesy of Wendie A. Berg, MD, PhD, FACR, Baltimore, MD. © Copyright 2006.)

mammography for lesions at the extremes of the superior, medial, inferior, or lateral breast. Lesions directly behind the nipple on both mammographic views will be directly behind the nipple on ultrasound. Careful angulation is necessary while performing ultrasound behind the nipple to avoid shadowing from the nipple-areolar complex. For lesions directly behind the nipple on mammography, there will be dramatic differences in measured distances from the nipple on ultrasound and mammography (Fig. 9), because the mammographic measurement is nearly entirely a measurement of depth from the skin surface/nipple to the lesion, but on ultrasound there will be a nearly "zero" horizontal distance from the nipple along the skin surface because the lesion is directly behind the nipple. With the supine position and gentle compression used in ultrasound, most breasts are 2 to 4 cm in total thickness (ie, depth; ACRIN 6666, www.acrin.org/currentprotocols/6666, unpublished observations), whereas there can easily be 10 to 13 cm from nipple to chest wall when the breast is positioned for mammography.

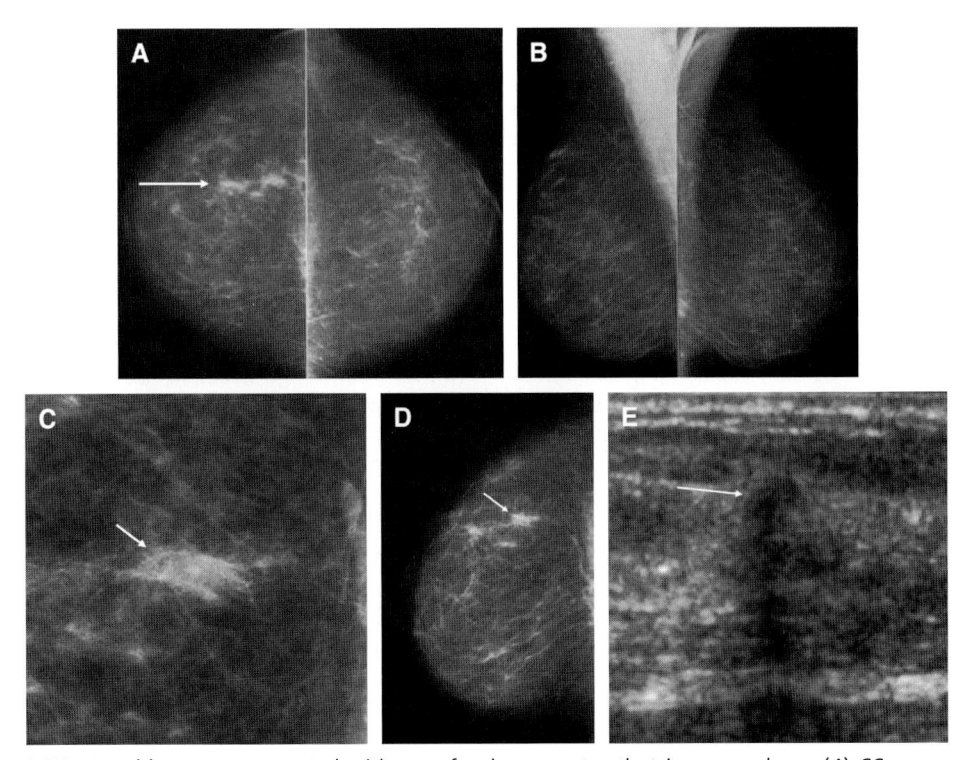

Fig. 4. A 74-year-old woman presented with new focal asymmetry that is seen only on (*A*) CC mammogram (*arrow*) and is not discrete on (*B*) MLO mammogram. (*C*) Spot-compression CC view confirms persistent indistinctly marginated mass (*arrow*). (*D*) On the CCRL view, the mass (*arrow*) moves laterally with the upper breast. (*E*) Transverse ultrasound at 12:00 in the right breast shows indistinctly marginated mass (*arrow*) with posterior shadowing. Ultrasound-guided biopsy showed invasive lobular carcinoma (ILC). (Case courtesy of Harmindar Gill, MD.) (Courtesy of Wendie A. Berg, MD, PhD, FACR, Baltimore, MD. © Copyright 2006.)

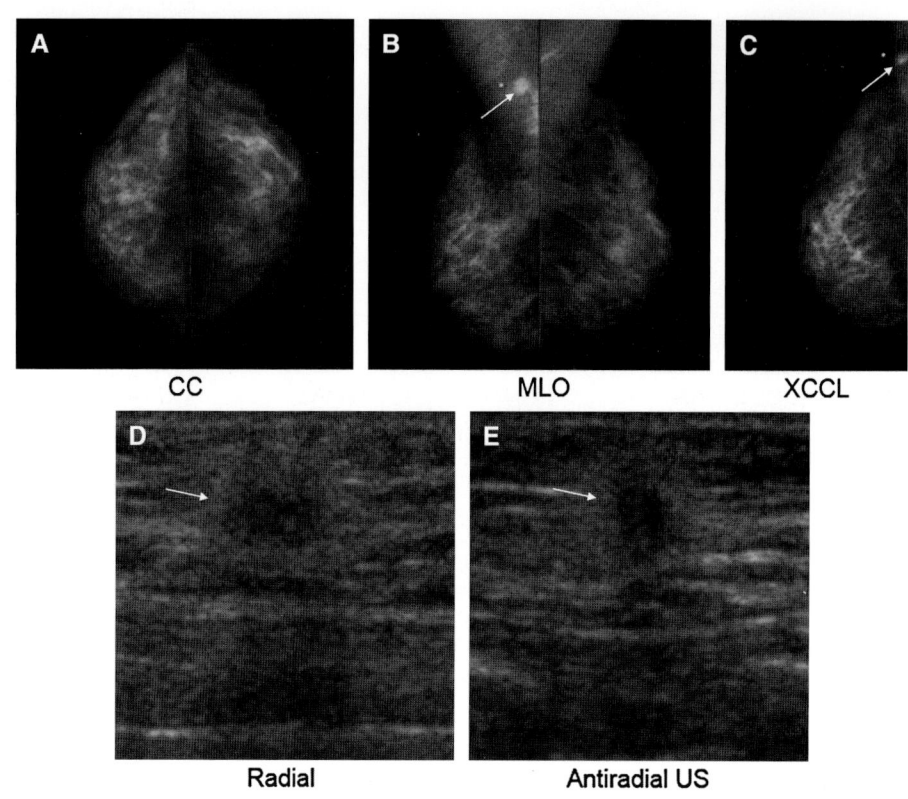

Fig. 5. A 44-year-old woman with a palpable mass right axilla. The mass is (*A*) occult on CC mammography and is seen only on (*B*) the MLO view (*arrow*). Such masses usually are located laterally, as confirmed on (*C*) the laterally exaggerated CC view (*arrow*). Targeted (*D*) radial and (*E*) antiradial ultrasound confirms an indistinctly margin-ated hypoechoic mass (*arrows*). Ultrasound-guided biopsy showed grade I infiltrating ductal carcinoma. (Courtesy of Wendie A. Berg, MD, PhD, FACR, Baltimore, MD. © Copyright 2006.)

Although it is desirable to identify lesions in both mammographic views, doing so is not always possible or required. Lesions in the extreme posterior medial breast may be difficult to include on the MLO view (Fig. 10). Similarly, lesions in the extreme posterior (see Figs. 8, 9) or posterolateral breast may be difficult to include fully on the CC view, although laterally exaggerated CC positioning usually will demonstrate posterolateral lesions (see Fig. 5). Because the relative position of most lesions often can be closely inferred from a single mammographic view (see Fig. 2), ultrasound can be targeted to such abnormalities successfully (see Fig. 10). A comprehensive ultrasound scan of the appropriate possible locations in the breast (eg, mirror-image clock-face locations such as 10:00 and 2:00) often suffice in such cases. If needed, as discussed later, a radiopaque marker (eg, a BB) can be placed over the lesion demonstrated on ultrasound, and an appropriate correlative repeat mammographic view can be obtained. If necessary, for lesions seen only on the CC mammogram, the breast can be scanned by supporting it with the patient in the sitting position to reproduce mammographic positioning more closely; this technique can be especially helpful for large breasts.

Use of intrinsic landmarks

Surrounding structures can be helpful in correlating mammographic and sonographic findings. For retroareolar masses (see Fig. 7), the nipple itself is such a landmark. A scar or known lesion can serve as such a landmark as well (Figs. 11, 12). Calcifying fat necrosis, cysts (Fig. 13), fibroadenomata, and occasionally intramammary lymph nodes can be useful as internal markers. The background tissue texture also should be considered: a lesion surrounded by fat mammographically also should be surrounded by fat on ultrasound. It should be noted that normal breast tissue has variable composition and echogenicity, with denser, more fibrotic tissue often more echogenic than subcutaneous fat. False-negative ultrasound examinations occasionally can occur with masses that are isoechoic to surrounding elements. Although occurring most commonly with benign lesions isoechoic to fat (eg, fibroadenomata [Fig. 14] or intramammary

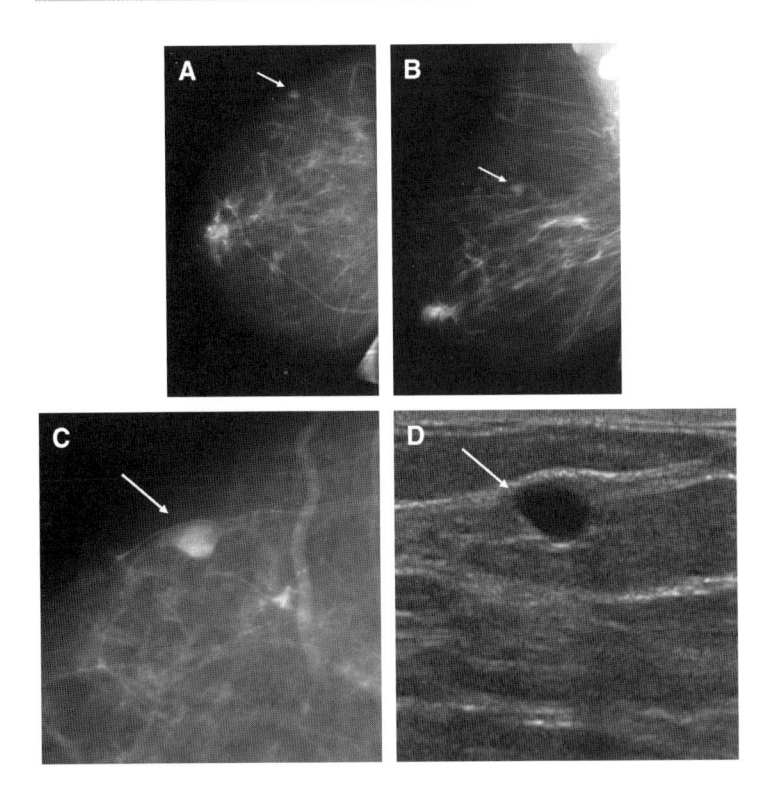

Fig. 6. A new nodule was noted in the outer right breast (*arrows*) in an 80-year-old woman receiving hormone replacement therapy. The mass moves inferiorly from (*A*) CC to (*B*) MLO views and is expected to be in the 9:00 position in the right breast and superficial (near the skin). (*C*) Spot-compression CC view confirms superficially located, mostly circumscribed oval mass (*arrow*). (*D*) Targeted ultrasound shows a superficial cyst (*arrow*) at the 9:30 position in the right breast, 8 cm from the nipple, corresponding in size, shape, and location with the mammographically depicted mass. Although it is posterior in the breast on mammography, the mass is superficial on ultrasound because it is near the skin. (Courtesy of Wendie A. Berg, MD, PhD, FACR, Baltimore, MD. © Copyright 2006.)

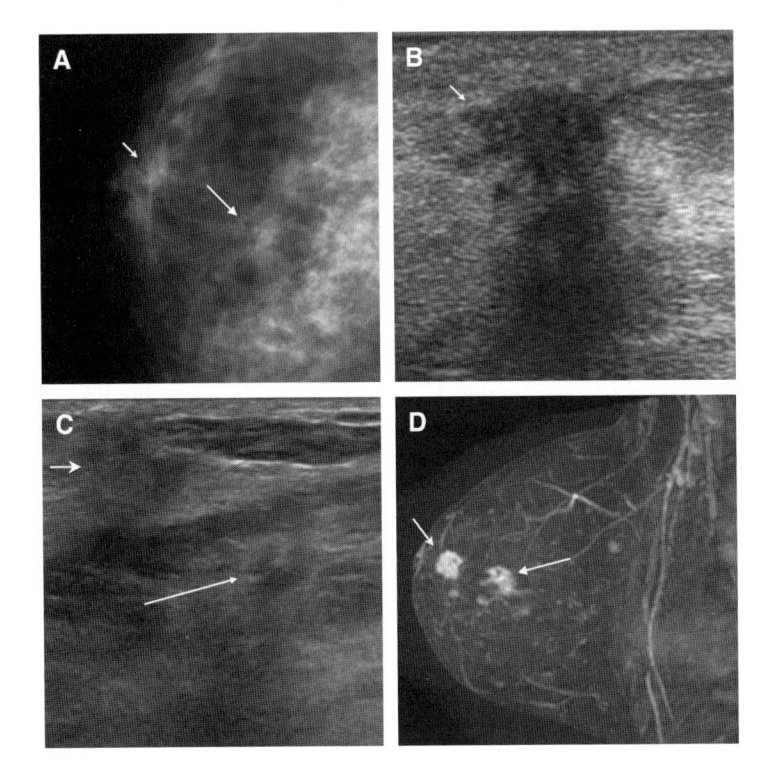

Fig. 7. This 44-year-old woman was noted to have two spiculated masses directly behind the nipple on mammography, seen best on (*A*) spot-compression CC view (*short arrow anteriorly; long arrow centrally*). (*B*) Initial transverse ultrasound showed speculated superficial mass (*short arrow*) at the nipple. The second mass could not initially be seen on ultrasound. (*C*) Second ultrasound performed with greater field of view shows the anterior mass (*short arrow*) as well as a subtle deeper irregular hypoechoic mass (*long arrow*) corresponding to the second mass seen more centrally on mammography. Both masses were biopsied under ultrasound guidance, showing in situ and infiltrating moderately differentiated carcinoma with predominantly lobular features. (*D*) The two masses are also well seen on contrast-enhanced MR imaging (*short arrow anteriorly; long arrow centrally*). (Courtesy of Wendie A. Berg, MD, PhD, FACR, Baltimore, MD. © Copyright 2006.)

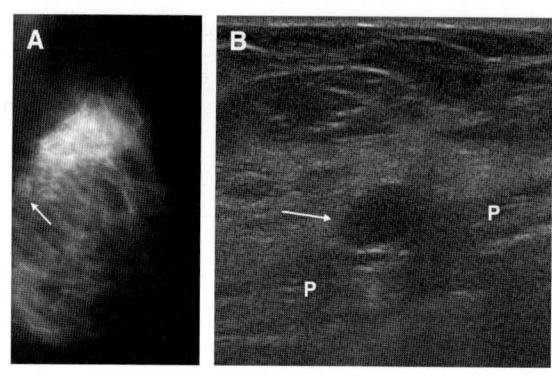

Fig. 8. (*A*) A 49-year-old woman with a new mass (*arrow*) in the posterior left breast on MLO only. (*B*) Radial ultrasound shows cyst (*arrow*) in the 3:30 position at chest wall. P, pectoral muscle. (Courtesy of Wendie A. Berg, MD, PhD, FACR, Baltimore, MD. © Copyright 2006.)

lymph nodes), ductal carcinoma in situ (DCIS) (see Fig. 13) and colloid (mucinous) carcinomas in particular can be isoechoic to fat [6,7] and occasionally can mimic the appearance of a fat lobule or be overlooked at sonography (Fig. 15).

Size

A small amount of magnification occurs with mammography in that most lesions are within the breast, with the amount of magnification increasing with increasing distance from the actual detector. Typically measurements on mammography should be no more than 20% larger than the diameter on ultrasound (Fig. 16). Malignancies on ultrasound may have an indistinct, gradual transition between lesion and tissue, often with a thick rim of surrounding echogenic desmoplasia; generally, the rim should not be included in the lesion measurements. Masses isoechoic to fat may be difficult to perceive and therefore to measure accurately (see Fig. 15). It may be particularly difficult to determine where to measure a mass with intraductal extension (Fig. 17). The intraductal component seen on ultrasound usually represents DCIS, which can be mammographically occult unless it is associated with calcifications (see Fig. 17). Measurement of the dominant mass component on ultrasound usually correlates best with the size of the pathologic invasive tumor size because DCIS is not included in pathologic measurements of tumor size per se. Although the DCIS component may not be measured optimally on ultrasound, knowledge of intraductal extension caused by DCIS can aid in preoperative planning by helping the surgeon include the DCIS component in the resected specimen and avoid positive margins [8,9]. Ultrasound is most accurate at sizing solitary invasive cancers 2 cm in size or smaller without an extensive intraductal component [9].

Masses

A mammographically discrete and probably circumscribed noncalcified mass on two views can proceed directly to further evaluation with

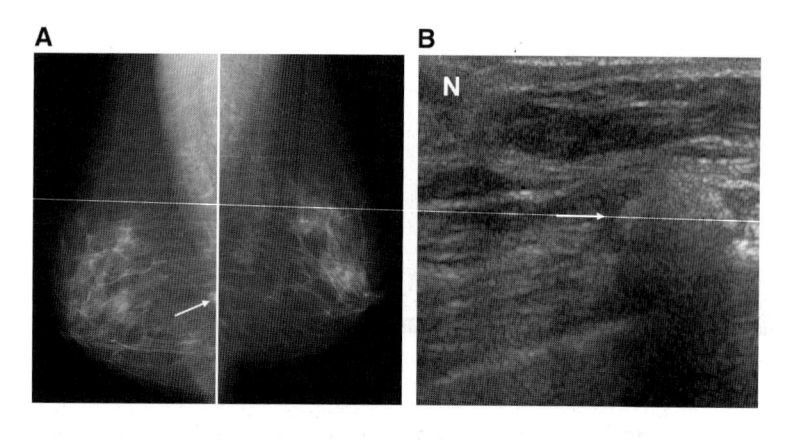

Fig. 9. (*A*) MLO mammogram shows circumscribed mass (*arrow*) at chest wall directly behind the nipple, which could not be included on laterally or medially exaggerated CC views, suggesting a central location. (*B*) Targeted ultrasound directly behind the nipple (N) shows corresponding snowstorm appearance of siliconoma (*arrow*) at the chest wall in this 58-year-old woman who has a history of implant removal. The distance from the nipple on mammography was 8 cm, compared with the horizontal 1- to 2-cm distance from the nipple along the skin surface on ultrasound. (Courtesy of Wendie A. Berg, MD, PhD, FACR, Baltimore, MD. © Copyright 2006.)

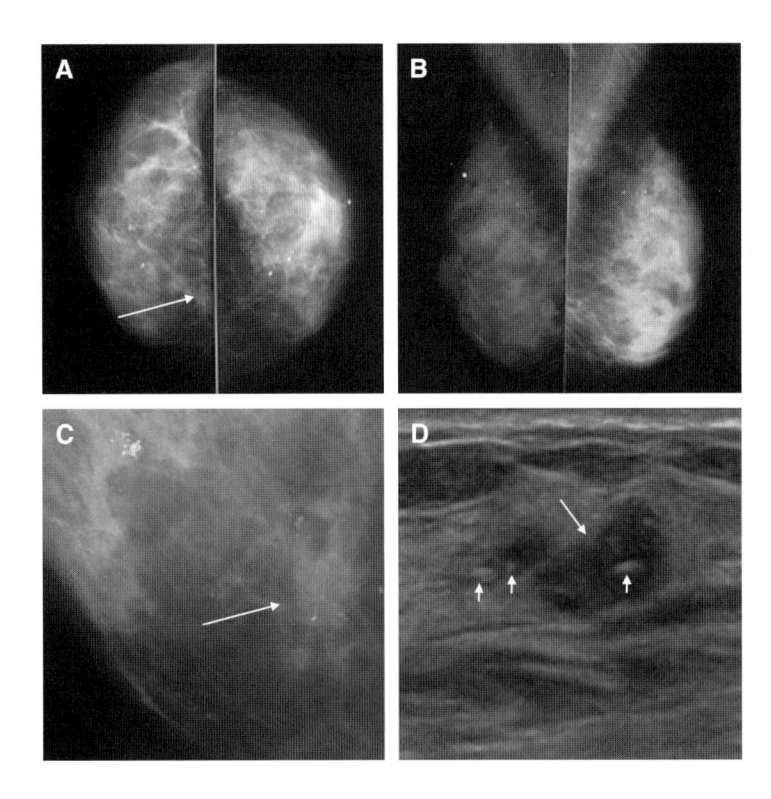

Fig. 10. A new spiculated mass with calcifications was noted in the extreme posterior-medial right breast in this 71-year-old woman, seen only on (*A*) CC view (*arrow*), occult on (*B*) MLO view, and confirmed on (*C*) spot-magnification CC view (*arrow*). (*D*) Radial ultrasound of the inner right breast showed an irregular hypoechoic mass (*arrow*) with calcifications (*arrowheads*) in the 2:30 position parasternally, believed to correspond to the mammographically depicted mass. Ultrasound-guided biopsy confirmed grade 2 invasive ductal carcinoma and DCIS. (Courtesy of Wendie A. Berg, MD, PhD, FACR, Baltimore, MD. © Copyright 2006.)

ultrasound if it is 8 mm or larger. The sonographic finding of a simple cyst (anechoic, circumscribed, imperceptible wall, and posterior enhancement) is a benign finding, with no further work-up required [10]. Ultrasound may not be able to reliably distinguish simple cysts from solid masses for lesions smaller than 8 mm [5]. Initial spot-compression or spot-magnification views are helpful in characterizing mass margins before ultrasound. For moderately or highly suspicious masses, particularly those that may contain calcifications, magnification CC and 90° lateral views are encouraged before ultrasound for better characterization of lesion morphology and to depict better the extent of potential malignancies. In the latter situation, the primary purpose of ultrasound is biopsy guidance (see Fig. 10). Ultrasound also can be used to evaluate mammographically occult multifocal, multicentric, or contralateral disease [8,11,12].

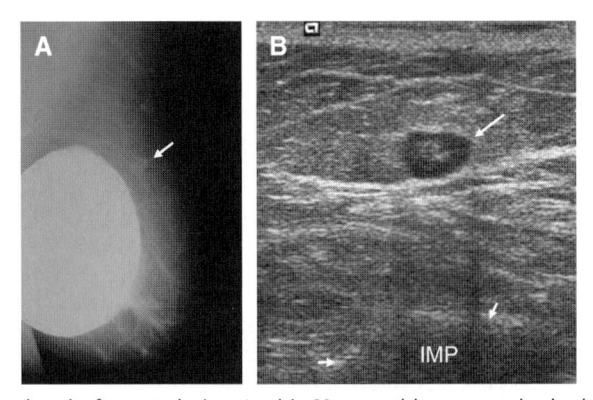

Fig. 11. Use of intrinsic landmarks for correlation. In this 60-year-old woman who had subglandular silicone implants for 33 years, an enlarging mass was noted adjacent to the left breast implant, seen only on (*A*) the MLO mammogram (*arrow*). (*B*) Ultrasound of the upper breast demonstrated a lymph node (*arrow*) adjacent to the implant (*arrowheads*, IMP) in the 2:00 position, 10 cm from the nipple. The size and location of the node relative to the nipple and the implant correlate well with the mammographic finding. (Courtesy of Wendie A. Berg, MD, PhD, FACR, Baltimore, MD. © Copyright 2006.)

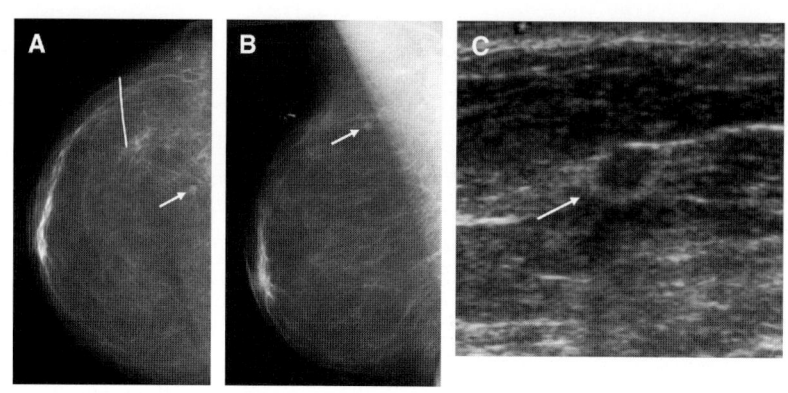

Fig. 12. Use of intrinsic landmarks. This 84-year-old woman had undergone lumpectomy 7 years earlier for cancer. A gradually enlarging mass (*arrows*) was noted near the lumpectomy scar on (*A*) CC and (*B*) MLO mammograms. (*C*) On ultrasound, with the scar used as a guide to location, a 4-mm microlobulated mass with echogenic halo was identified (*arrow*). Ultrasound-guided core biopsy showed grade I infiltrating ductal carcinoma. (Courtesy of Wendie A. Berg, MD, PhD, FACR, Baltimore, MD. © Copyright 2006.)

In addition to the location and size of the mass to be targeted, its morphology should be considered when correlating mammographic and sonographic findings. The American College of Radiology's Breast Imaging Reporting and Data System lexicons for mammography [1] and ultrasound [13] provide similar descriptors for most key mass features. A spiculated mass on mammography should be identifiable on ultrasound as an irregular, usually hypoechoic, spiculated mass, often with posterior shadowing and an echogenic rim or halo; ultrasound then can be used to guide biopsy. Radial scars usually are more subtle than carcinomas on ultrasound; in one recent series only 43% of radial scars were seen on ultrasound, compared with 93% of carcinomas [14]. Excision is recommended after a core biopsy diagnosis of a radial scar or a radial sclerosing lesion manifest as a mass or distortion, because of the risk of adjacent unsampled malignancy [15].

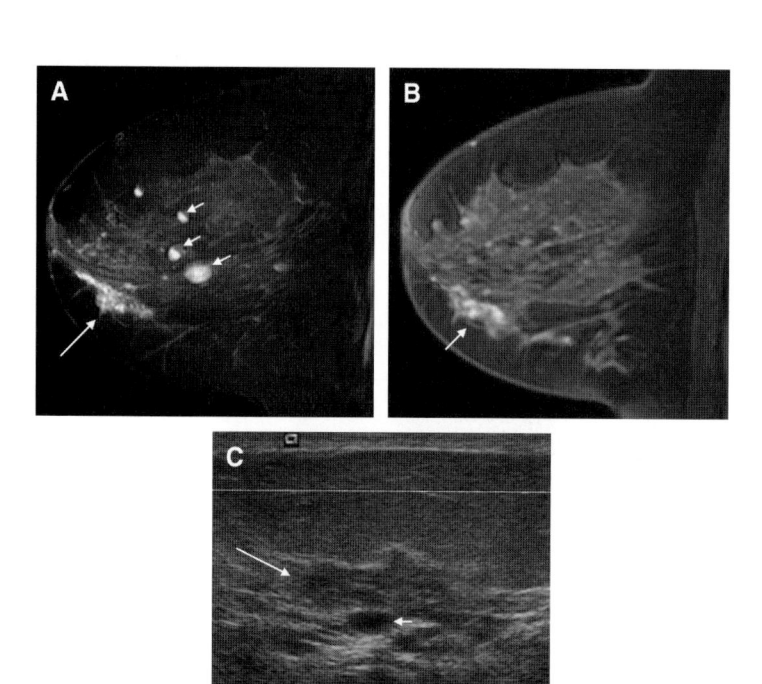

Fig. 13. DCIS can be quite subtle on ultrasound, as in this 47-year-old woman. (*A*) Inversion recovery MR imaging shows segment of increased signal retroareolar left breast 6:00 (*arrow*) as well as several adjacent cysts (*arrowheads*). (*B*) Sagittal T1-weighted spoiled gradient recalled (TR5/TE1.9) image 1.5 minutes after intravenous injection of 0.1 mmol/kg Gadolinium-diethylenetriamine pentaacetic acid shows segmental clumped enhancement in the 6:00 retroareolar left breast (*arrows*). (*C*) Ultrasound targeted to the MR imaging abnormality shows an isoechoic tubular mass (*arrow*) shown to be intermediate-grade DCIS on ultrasound-guided core biopsy. Adjacent (deeper) cysts are noted (*arrowheads*). (Courtesy of Wendie A. Berg, MD, PhD, FACR, Baltimore, MD. © Copyright 2006.)

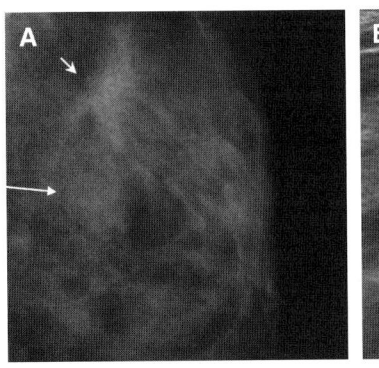

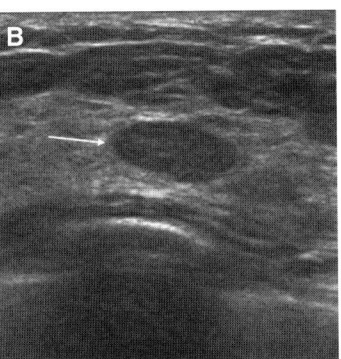

Fig. 14. Isoechoic masses can be difficult to see on ultrasound. (*A*) Spot-compression MLO mammogram demonstrates a spiculated mass (*short arrow*) known to be invasive lobular cancer in this 56-year-old woman. (*B*) An adjacent oval, partially circumscribed, partially obscured mass (*long arrow*) resembling a fat lobule was found to be an isoechoic, subtle mass on ultrasound. Ultrasound-guided core biopsy confirmed fibroadenoma. (Courtesy of Wendie A. Berg, MD, PhD, FACR, Baltimore, MD. © Copyright 2006.)

An indistinctly marginated mass on mammography is suspicious for malignancy, with 44% of such masses proving malignant in the series of Liberman and colleagues [16]. A spectrum of benign and malignant lesions can appear indistinct on mammography and yet be clearly benign on ultrasound (Fig. 18). Some masses that are thought to be circumscribed but are partially obscured by overlying tissue on mammography may actually prove indistinct or even spiculated on ultrasound

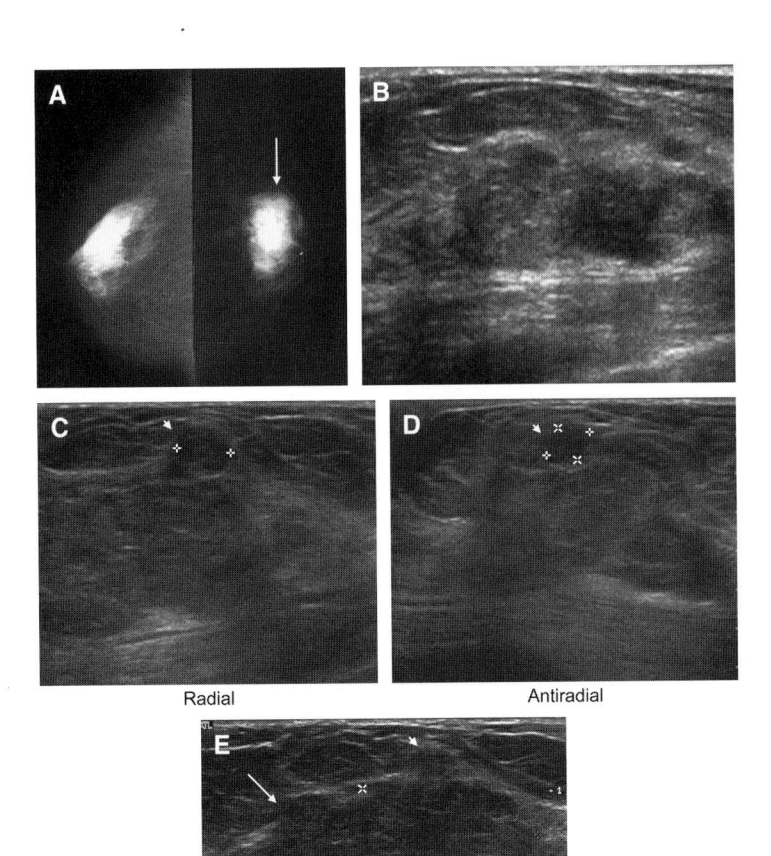

Fig. 15. Isoechoic malignancies can be a source of false-negative ultrasound. This 73-year-old woman had dense, nodular breast tissue for 25 years. (*A*) CC mammograms show symmetric dense tissue, although a longstanding palpable abnormality was noted in the left breast (*arrow*). (*B*) The initial ultrasound of the left breast was interpreted as negative, showing heterogeneous echotexture. On follow-up (*C*) radial and (*D*) antiradial ultrasound 6 months later, the technologist initially marked an 8-mm mass (*arrowheads, calipers*). (*E*) Re-evaluation ultrasound showed a 4.4 × 1.9 × 3.4 cm isoechoic lobulated mass (*arrow, marked by calipers*). Ultrasound-guided biopsy showed colloid (mucinous) carcinoma, which measured 4.5 cm at excision. The small anterior component of the mass, originally interpreted as the entire finding, is again marked (*arrowhead*). (Courtesy of Wendie A. Berg, MD, PhD, FACR, Baltimore, MD. © Copyright 2006.)

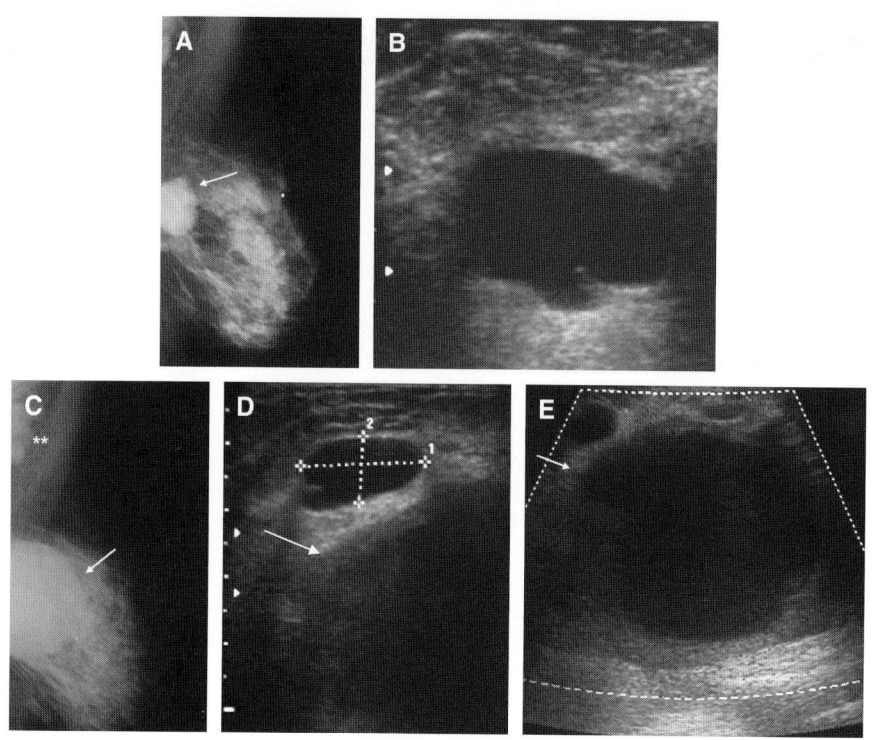

Fig. 16. Size discrepancy. (*A*) This 47-year-old woman noted a lump in the upper outer left breast, shown to correspond to a 3.5-cm dense mass on MLO mammogram (*arrow*). (*B*) Ultrasound (*right image*) showed a 1.4-cm cyst in this area; the finding was dismissed as benign. (*C*) Follow-up mammogram 12 months later shows the palpable mass enlarging, now 7 cm in size (*arrow*), with suspicious axillary nodes noted (******). (*D*) On follow-up ultrasound the 14-mm cyst is again seen (*calipers*), now noted to be at the anterior aspect of a 6.5-cm thick-walled cystic mass (*arrow*), caused by grade 3 invasive ductal carcinoma. (*E*) The mass is seen better on large field of view ultrasound. The large cancer was missed on the original ultrasound examination because the inadequate field of view did not include the posterior tissues. For concordance of mammographic and sonographic findings, the diameter on mammography usually should not be more than 20% larger than the diameter on ultrasound. In this case the large size discrepancy (3.5 cm on mammography versus 1.4 cm on ultrasound) was well beyond such thresholds. (Courtesy of Wendie A. Berg, MD, PhD, FACR, Baltimore, MD. © Copyright 2006.)

(Fig. 19). Because of the inherently different physics of the respective modalities, elements with a similar mammographic density can have vastly different acoustic transmission and thus often can be exquisitely resolved with ultrasound. Indeed, supplemental lesion detection with ultrasound is of potentially greatest value in mammographically dense parenchyma [17].

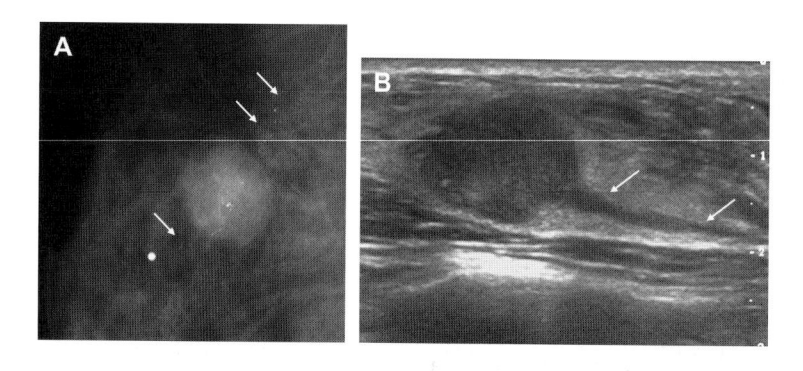

Fig. 17. (*A*) A palpable mass and adjacent segmental calcifications (*arrows*) seen on MLO mammography in a 44-year-old woman. (*B*) The intraductal extension (*arrows*) seen on ultrasound is important to document, because it typically represents DCIS, and preoperative documentation of the intraductal extension facilitates achieving clear margins. The invasive component usually is limited to the dominant mass, as in this case of a 2.8-cm grade 3 infiltrating ductal carcinoma with associated DCIS. (Courtesy of Wendie A. Berg, MD, PhD, FACR, Baltimore, MD. © Copyright 2006.)

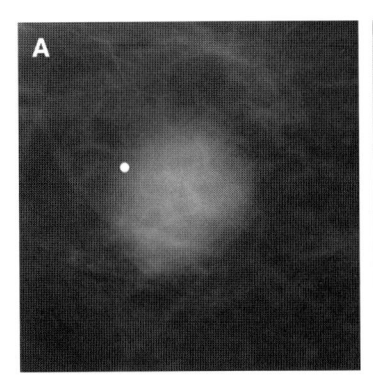

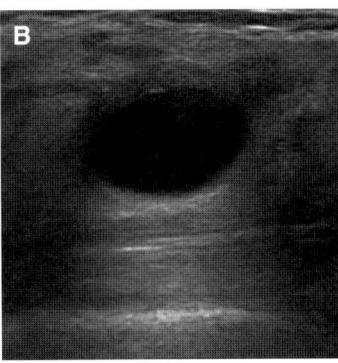

Fig. 18. A 46-year-old woman with a palpable mass. (*A*) Spot-compression CC mammogram shows an indistinctly margin-ated palpable mass. (*B*) Antiradial ultrasound shows mass to correspond to a simple cyst. (Courtesy of Wendie A. Berg, MD, PhD, FACR, Baltimore, MD. © Copyright 2006.)

One of the greatest challenges in correlating mammographic and sonographic findings is the patient who has multiple, bilateral, partially circumscribed, partially obscured masses. In general, such findings can be considered benign, with the risk of malignancy less than in the general screening population [18], with no need for ultrasound evaluation. Each mass must be evaluated carefully, however; any mass that appears indistinctly marginated or otherwise of concern merits further evaluation with ultrasound and possibly additional mammographic views. Even though most fluctuating, mostly circumscribed bilateral masses are caused by cysts or fibroadenomas, ultrasound is needed for evaluation of a dominant or clinically suspicious mass in this setting (Fig. 20). When multiple, bilateral, similar-appearing, oval, circumscribed, solid masses are seen on ultrasound, the assumption is that these masses are probably benign and can be followed at 6 months; further validation of this approach is in progress (www.acrin.org/currentprotocols/ACRIN6666) [17].

Having an appropriate preliminary differential based on the initial mammographic assessment is critical. Although quite complementary, mammography and ultrasound each has strengths and limitations. For instance, should the preliminary mammographic assessment of a nodule suggest that it might represent an intramammary node, one must keep in mind that these nodes can be quite subtle sonographically. At ultrasound, normal lymph nodes often blend in with surrounding parenchyma (Fig. 21), although reactive and metastatic nodes often have a hypoechoic or anechoic, thickened cortex and a diminutive hilum (with the cortex most often symmetrically thickened in reactive nodes and more commonly asymmetrically thickened in metastatic nodes) [19]. Spot-compression or magnification mammographic views often are more helpful than ultrasound in characterizing a circumscribed mass suspected to be a (normal) lymph node; the reniform shape of the node can be seen when the fatty hilum is in profile (Fig. 22).

Asymmetries and architectural distortion

When evaluating asymmetries, comparison with prior mammograms may demonstrate stability and preclude the need for further workup. Sickles [20] found one-view asymmetries present on approximately 3% of screening mammograms; in more than half of these, the finding could be

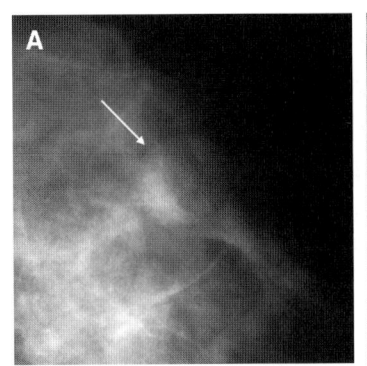

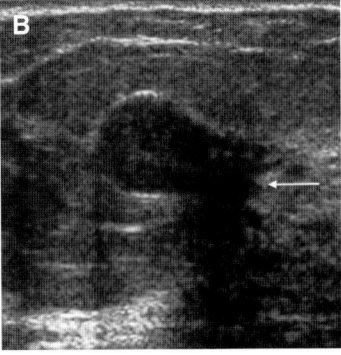

Fig. 19. (*A*) A 40-year-old woman with a partially obscured nodule (*arrow*) noted on baseline screening (close-up of CC view). (*B*) Transverse ultrasound demonstrates mostly circumscribed, partially irregular hypoechoic mass (*arrow*) corresponding to the mammographic abnormality. Biopsy showed fibroadenoma involved by ILC and lobular carcinoma in situ. (Courtesy of Wendie A. Berg, MD, PhD, FACR, Baltimore, MD. © Copyright 2006.)

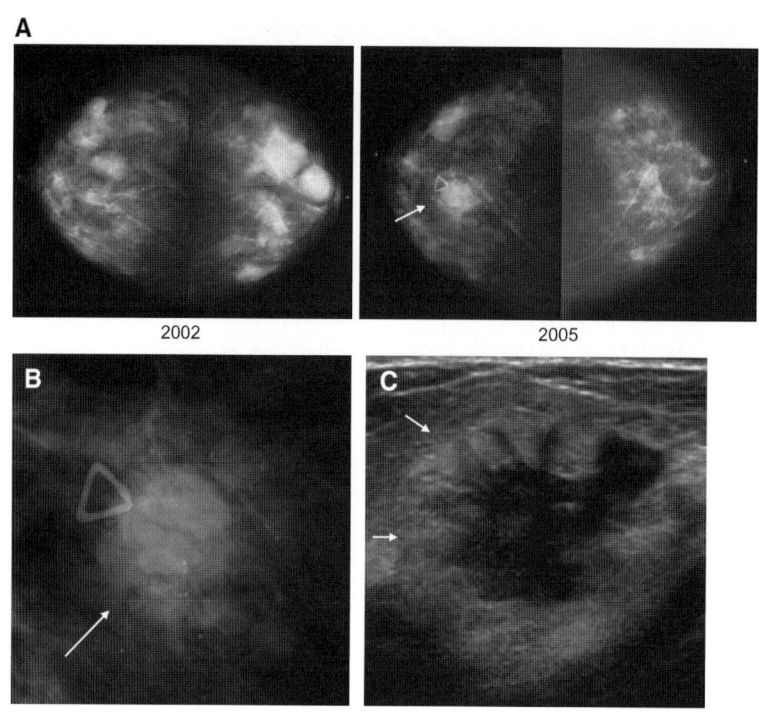

Fig. 20. A 68-year-old woman with known cysts. (*A*) Mammographically, there were multiple bilateral, mostly circumscribed masses, some developing and others regressing compared with prior mammogram obtained 3 years earlier (*left image*). One dominant, palpable mass (*arrow*), marked by skin marker, was currently noted in the right breast. (*B*) On the spot-compression CC view, the margins of the palpable mass can be seen to be spiculated (*arrow*). (*C*) Ultrasound of the palpable mass confirms spiculated margins and hyperechoic rim (*short arrows*). Ultrasound-guided biopsy and excision showed poorly differentiated invasive ductal carcinoma. Although multiple, bilateral circumscribed masses usually are benign, careful attention should be directed to the margins of each mass, and ultrasound is appropriate for any suspicious mass and/or any dominant or palpable mass. (*Courtesy of Wendie A. Berg, MD, PhD, FACR, Baltimore, MD.* © *Copyright 2006.*)

dismissed as summation shadow from the screening views alone [20]. Asymmetries are a frequent cause of overlooked malignancy [21]. New focal asymmetries usually require additional mammographic evaluation before ultrasound and carry an approximately 20% risk of malignancy [22]. Spot-compression views help confirm persistence of an underlying mass and often depict mass margins better than do routine mammographic views (see Figs. 4, 23).

Normal variant asymmetry lacks calcifications or distortion, contains interspersed fat on mammography, and often correlates with echogenic fibroglandular elements on ultrasound (Figs. 24, 25). Clear concordance in size, morphology, and location often can be exquisitely demonstrated with

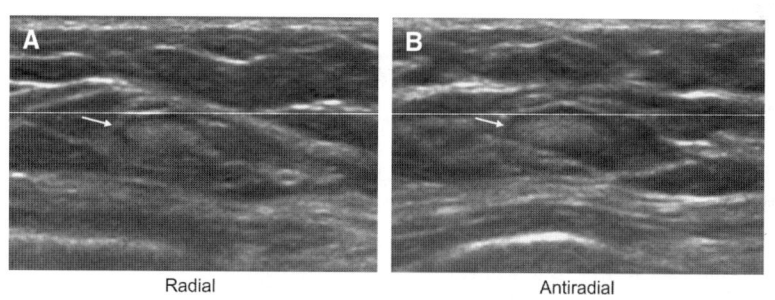

Fig. 21. Normal lymph nodes can blend in with the surrounding parenchyma on ultrasound, as in this 60-year-old woman. On (*A*) radial, and (*B*) antiradial ultrasound, note thin cortex (*arrows*), slightly hypo- to isoechoic to surrounding fat, and central echogenic fatty hilum. (*Courtesy of Wendie A. Berg, MD, PhD, FACR, Baltimore, MD.* © *Copyright 2006.*)

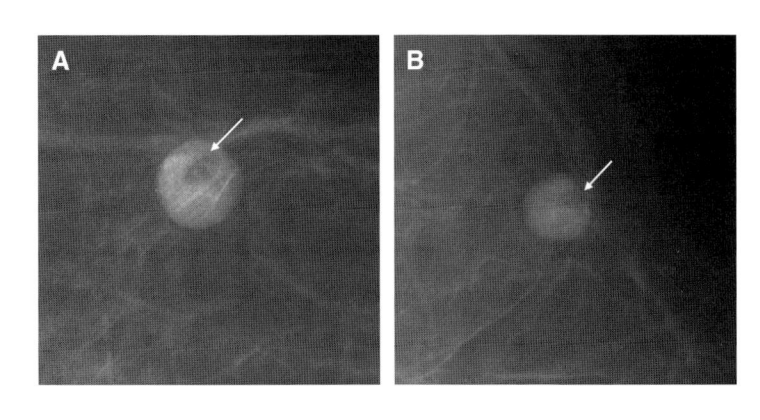

Fig. 22. Close-ups of (*A*) CC and (*B*) MLO mammograms show circumscribed nodule containing fat (*arrows*). The reniform shape is appreciated better on the MLO view. Note the close proximity to vessels that feed the hilum, as is often demonstrated on color or power Doppler ultrasound. Findings are characteristic of a benign lymph node. (Courtesy of Wendie A. Berg, MD, PhD, FACR, Baltimore, MD. © Copyright 2006.)

ultrasound, confirming that the asymmetry represents a normal variant. In current practice, such typical findings generally would preclude biopsy, particularly if the asymmetry is nonpalpable. If sampled, stromal fibrosis or atrophic breast tissue would be concordant results (see Fig. 25).

Invasive lobular carcinoma (ILC), in particular, can manifest as a focal asymmetry, often on only one mammographic view, more often the CC view (see Fig. 4). Spot-compression views may reveal associated architectural distortion. Ultrasound can be particularly helpful in depicting mammographically subtle or occult ILC [8,23], although the findings can be quite subtle (Figs. 26,27). The size of ILC often is underestimated on both mammography and ultrasound [24], particularly for tumors larger than 3 cm in size. MR imaging is particularly helpful in depicting and characterizing the extent of ILC [25,26].

Absence of a sonographic correlate should not deter further evaluation or biopsy in the setting of an unexplained new focal asymmetry [27] or distortion. MR imaging can be helpful in further evaluation in this setting [28]. Importantly, apparent thinning of a focal asymmetry on spot-compression views does not necessarily preclude further evaluation with ultrasound if the initial finding was suspicious; the same concept applies to architectural distortion (Fig. 28).

Architectural distortion on mammography should be seen as tethering of Cooper's ligaments on ultrasound (see Fig. 27). Ultrasound can reveal an underlying mass (see Fig. 27) and be used to guide biopsy. Postsurgical scars are a common

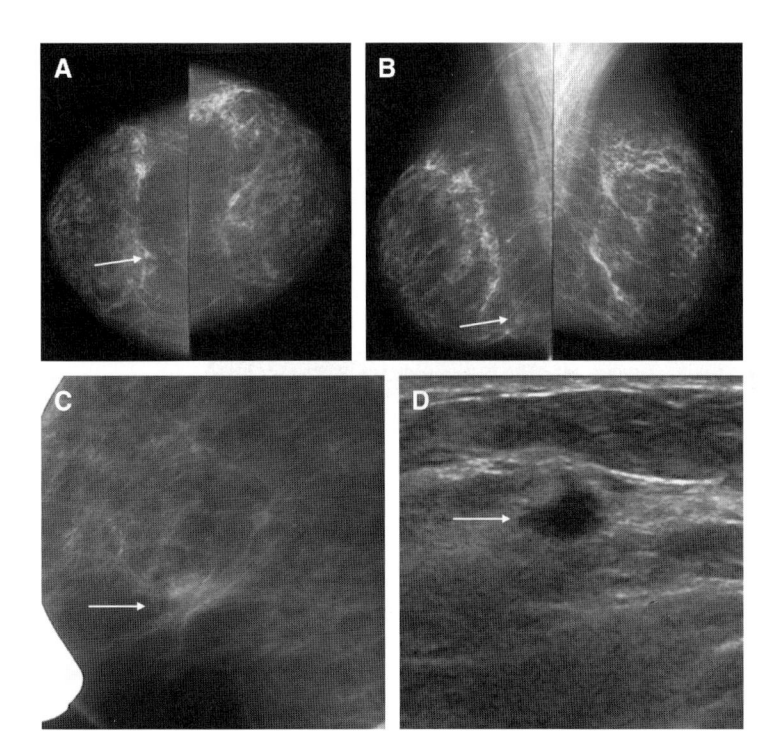

Fig. 23. New focal asymmetry was noted on annual screening mammograms in the lower inner right breast posteriorly on (*A*) CC and (*B*) MLO mammograms (*arrows*) in this 62-year-old woman. (*C*) Spot-compression MLO view better depicts an indistinctly marginated mass (*arrow*). (*D*) Antiradial ultrasound targeted to the mammographic abnormality, at 5:00 in the right breast, shows an indistinctly marginated mass (*arrow*) of the same shape and size. Ultrasound-guided biopsy showed grade 2 invasive ductal carcinoma. (Courtesy of Wendie A. Berg, MD, PhD, FACR, Baltimore, MD. © Copyright 2006.)

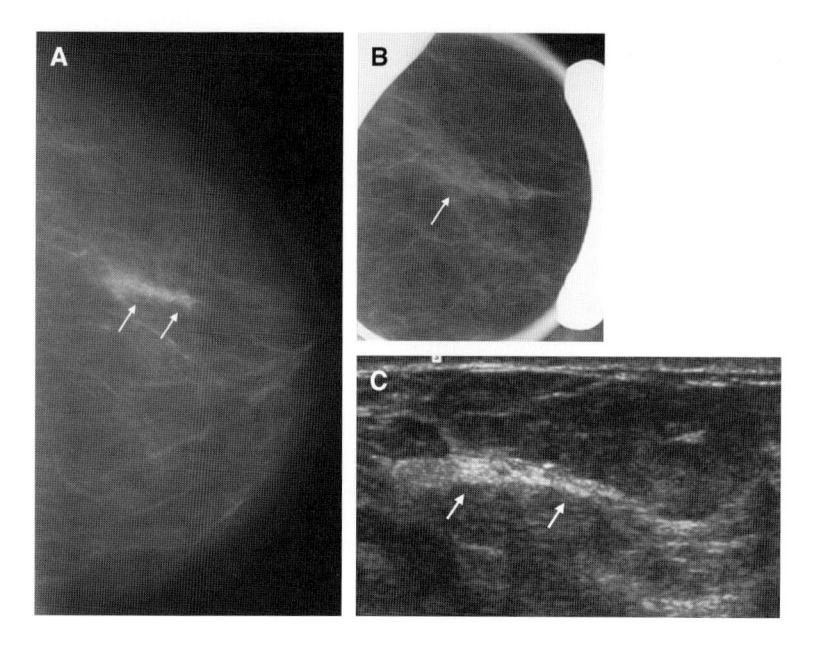

Fig. 24. Bandlike asymmetry is noted on (*A*) CC mammogram (*arrows*), which partially thins on (*B*) spot-compression CC mammograms (*arrows*) and appears to contain interspersed fat. (*C*) Targeted ultrasound revealed a homogeneously hyperechoic band of tissue (*arrows*), correlating in size and location with the mammographic abnormality. The ultrasound appearance is typical of normal variant fibrotic tissue. (Courtesy of Wendie A. Berg, MD, PhD, FACR, Baltimore, MD. © Copyright 2006.)

cause of distortion (Fig. 29). On ultrasound, in addition to distortion, a hypoechoic, area, often with shadowing, is commonly seen, and it should be possible on ultrasound to depict the track to the overlying skin incision site where there is usually associated skin thickening (> 2 mm; see Fig. 29) and occasionally even skin retraction. The scar itself generally should be concave once any associated fluid collection has resolved and should continue to decrease over time, as has been described on mammography [29].

Calcifications

Many believe ultrasound does not contribute significantly to the assessment of indeterminate calcifications. Although not of value in further characterization of the morphology or the extent of calcifications per se [30], ultrasound can prove useful in the evaluation of suspected DCIS. At times, a clear sonographic correlate can be identified if involved ducts are distended with tumor or necrotic debris with or without calcifications (Figs. 30, 31). When visualized sonographically, DCIS can be biopsied under ultrasound guidance. Ultrasound can rarely help depict unexpected duct extension toward the nipple or demonstrate multifocality or multicentricity of DCIS [8,31], although MR imaging is more accurate in this context [8,32,33].

The existence of a sonographic correlate to suspicious calcifications has important implications. Soo

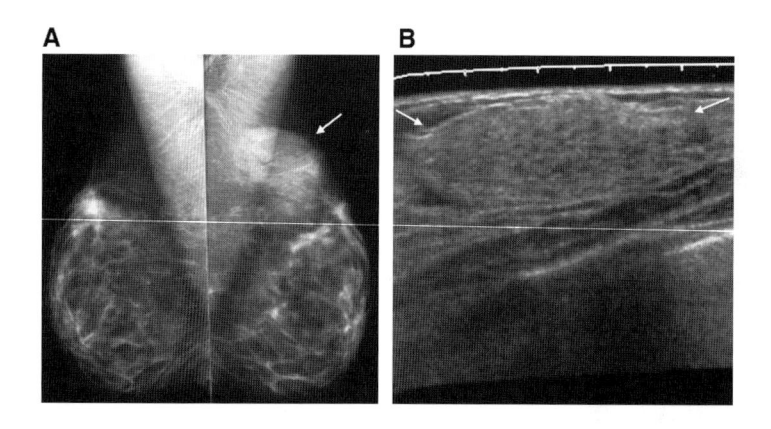

Fig. 25. MLO mammograms in this 47-year-old woman show (*A*) global asymmetry in the axillary tail of the left breast (*arrow*). (*B*) Ultrasound targeted to the asymmetry demonstrates an ovoid area of increased echogenicity (*arrows*). Tiny hypoechoic areas represent residual fat and/or terminal duct lobular units. The appearance is consistent with normal variant fibrotic tissue. Because the area was vaguely palpable, ultrasound-guided core biopsy was performed, confirming stromal fibrosis. (Courtesy of Wendie A. Berg, MD, PhD, FACR, Baltimore, MD. © Copyright 2006.)

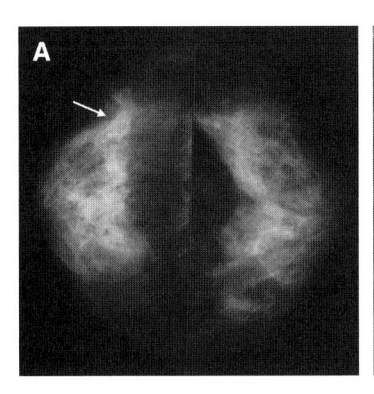

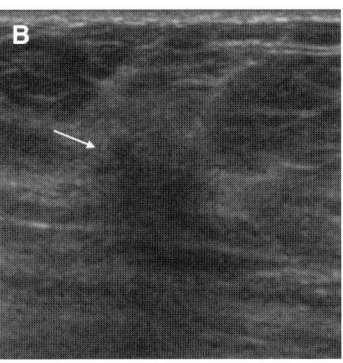

Fig. 26. Architectural distortion was noted in the outer right breast in this 56-year-old woman, seen best on (*A*) CC mammogram (*arrow*). (*B*) Radial ultrasound of the outer right breast in the 10:00 position showed a subtle hypoechoic irregular mass (*arrow*). Ultrasound-guided core biopsy showed invasive lobular carcinoma. (Courtesy of Wendie A. Berg, MD, PhD, FACR, Baltimore, MD. © Copyright 2006.)

and colleagues [34] performed ultrasound on a consecutive series of 111 lesions of suspicious calcifications going to biopsy and were able to depict 26 (23%) on ultrasound. In a similar series, Moon and colleagues [35] depicted 45% of 100 mammographically detected clustered calcifications on ultrasound, with all malignancies larger than 10 mm seen as masses on ultrasound. In the series of Soo and colleagues [34], also, the lesions seen on ultrasound were larger than those not seen, had more calcifications, and were seen as masses (77%) (see Fig. 31) or dilated ducts (23%) containing echogenic foci (see Fig. 30) [34]. Calcifications seen on ultrasound were more likely in malignant lesions (69% versus 21%); when malignant calcifications were identified on ultrasound, the calcifications were more likely to be associated with invasive than in situ carcinoma [34]. Thus, in the setting of a broad area of mammographically suspicious calcifications likely to be DCIS, ultrasound can help identify the associated invasive component, if any, and thereby help guide treatment planning (Fig. 32). The absence of a sonographic correlate for mammographically suspicious calcifications should not preclude biopsy, because more than half of DCIS cases may be sonographically occult [8].

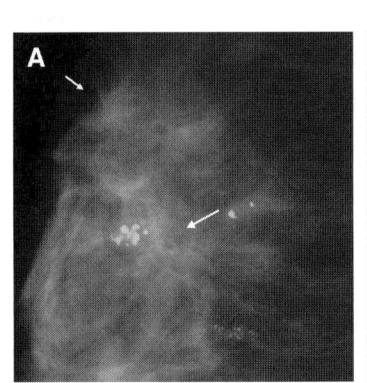

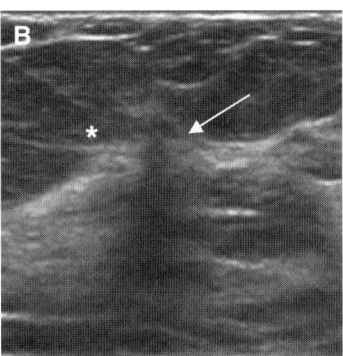

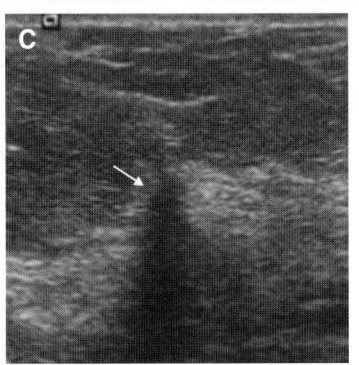

Fig. 27. Multifocal invasive lobular carcinoma. (*A*) Spot-magnification mediolateral view in this 56-year-old woman demonstrates subtle architectural distortion (*long arrow*) and adjacent spiculated mass (*short arrow*). (*B*) Initial ultrasound showed a solitary, vertically oriented hypoechoic mass (*long arrow*) with associated posterior shadowing, distortion, and tethering of Cooper ligaments (***), which proved to be at the site of mammographic distortion. Ultrasound-guided core biopsy showed ILC. (*C*) Repeat ultrasound of the surrounding tissue the following week demonstrated an adjacent irregular hypoechoic mass (*short arrow*) with posterior shadowing. Ultrasound-guided biopsy confirmed multifocal ILC. Clips (not shown) proved the second mass to correspond to the more superior spiculated mass shown on mammography. (Courtesy of Wendie A. Berg, MD, PhD, FACR, Baltimore, MD. © Copyright 2006.)

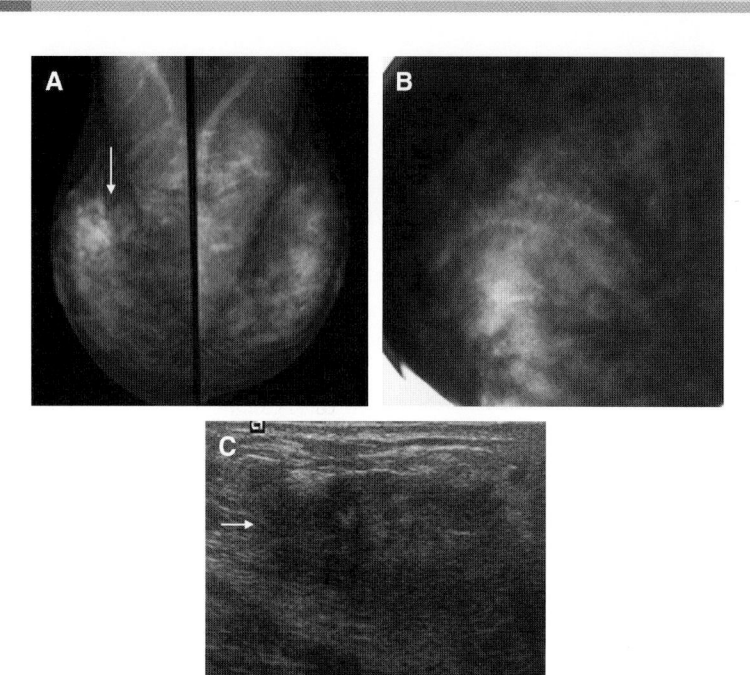

Fig. 28. A 52-year-old woman was recalled for architectural distortion noted on (*A*) screening MLO mammogram of the upper right breast (*arrow*). (*B*) On spot-compression MLO, the area was thought to thin and was dismissed. Four months later nipple retraction was noted. (*C*) Ultrasound at that time depicted a 6-cm underlying irregular hypoechoic mass (*arrow*) centered in the same area as the distortion (ie, at 10:00 in the right breast). Ultrasound-guided core biopsy showed ILC. (Courtesy of Wendie A. Berg, MD, PhD, FACR, Baltimore, MD. © Copyright 2006.)

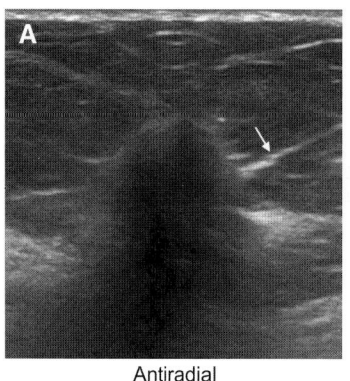

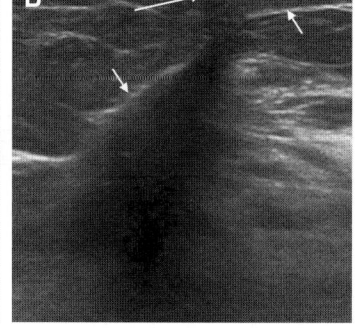

Fig. 29. Postsurgical scar. Four years after lumpectomy for cancer at this site, (*A*) antiradial and (*B*) radial ultrasound images show an area of decreased echogenicity and posterior shadowing with associated tethering of Cooper ligaments (*short arrows*). On the radial image, the track to overlying skin scar is evident, with associated skin thickening (*long arrow*), compatible with a postsurgical scar. (Courtesy of Wendie A. Berg, MD, PhD, FACR, Baltimore, MD. © Copyright 2006.)

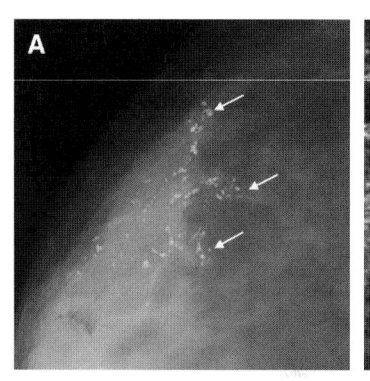

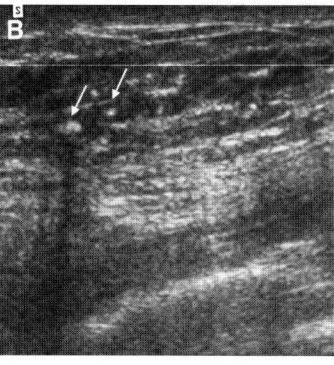

Fig. 30. An 84-year-old woman with contralateral invasive ductal cancer. (*A*) Magnification MLO view shows segmental pleomorphic and coarse heterogeneous calcifications (*arrows*). (*B*) Targeted ultrasound shows distended ducts containing echogenic foci (*arrows*) due to calcifications. Ultrasound-guided biopsy showed high-grade DCIS. (Courtesy of Wendie A. Berg, MD, PhD, FACR, Baltimore, MD. © Copyright 2006.)

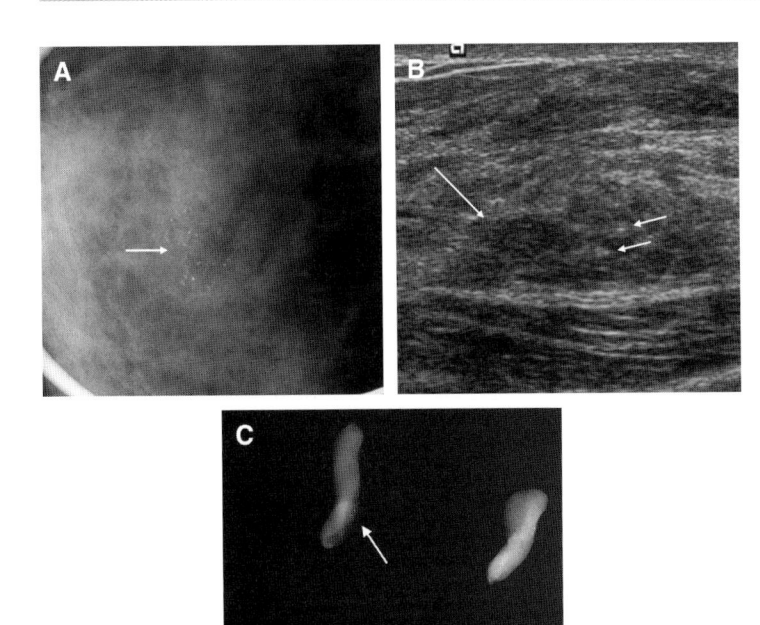

Fig. 31. (*A*) CC magnification view in this 40-year-old woman shows regional pleomorphic calcifications (*arrow*) in the right breast as noted on baseline screening. (*B*) Targeted ultrasound shows a 2.5-cm ill-defined mass (*long arrow*) with a few echogenic calcifications. Ten-gauge vacuum-assisted biopsy was performed under ultrasound guidance. (*C*) Specimen radiograph confirms retrieval of calcifications (*arrow*). Histopathology showed high-grade DCIS. (Courtesy of Wendie A. Berg, MD, PhD, FACR, Baltimore, MD. © Copyright 2006.)

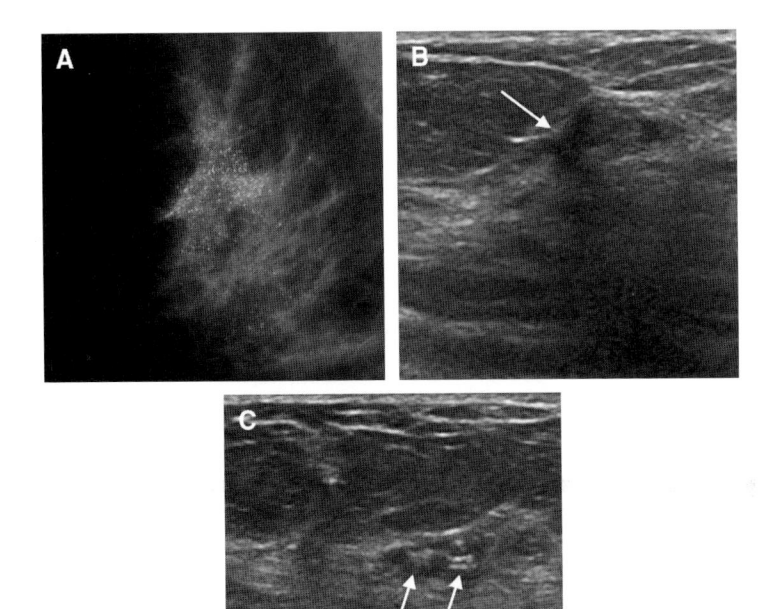

Fig. 32. (*A*) A 47-year-old woman with extensive segmental pleomorphic calcifications on MLO mammography. (*B*) Ultrasound showed a solitary 9-mm spiculated mass (*arrow*) as well as (*C*) numerous echogenic foci compatible with calcifications, some of which were clearly intraductal (*arrows*). Ultrasound-guided core biopsy of the mass in B showed high-grade invasive ductal carcinoma. At surgery, 1.2-cm invasive ductal carcinoma with extensive high-grade DCIS was found. Ultrasound can help depict an invasive component preoperatively. When there is known invasive tumor, axillary lymph node(s) are sampled. Further, the pathologist can miss such a small invasive component when the mastectomy specimen is examined. Sampling the mass under ultrasound guidance (with clip placement) facilitates both preoperative planning and evaluation of the mastectomy specimen. (Courtesy of Wendie A. Berg, MD, PhD, FACR, Baltimore, MD. © Copyright 2006.)

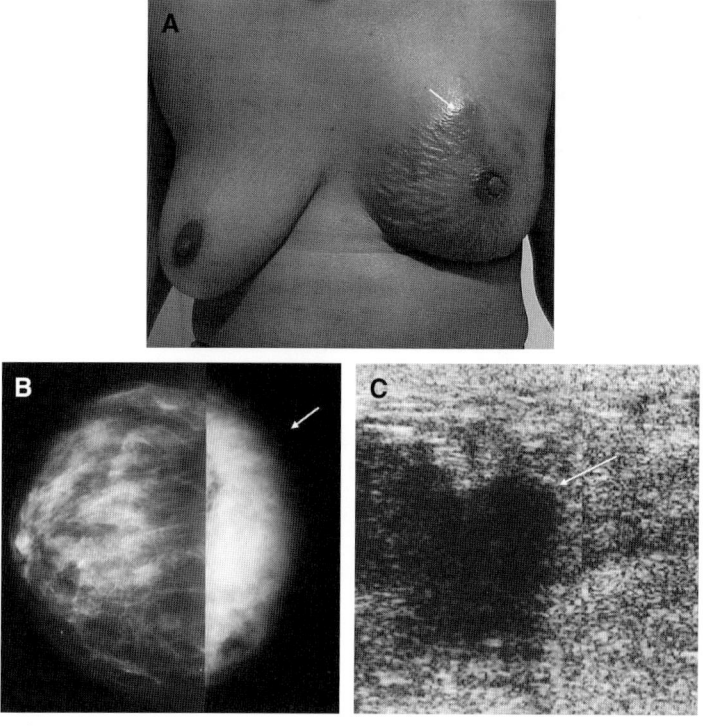

Fig. 33. (*A*) Erythema, hardening, nipple retraction, and diffuse skin thickening with palpable cords were noted in the left breast of this 43-year-old woman. The skin-punch biopsy site is marked (*arrow*) but was nondiagnostic. (*B*) Only CC mammograms could be performed and demonstrate diffuse increased density on the left side (*arrow*). Ultrasound-guided biopsy was requested. (*C*) In the 3:00 axis, an irregular, hypoechoic mass was identified (*arrow*). Diffuse increased echogenicity caused by edema is noted in the surrounding parenchyma. A skin incision was made where the skin was normal, and an ultrasound-guided 14-gauge core biopsy was performed, yielding poorly differentiated infiltrating mammary carcinoma with lymphovascular invasion. This case is a variant of inflammatory carcinoma in which the breast appears shrunken, mimicking ILC, rather than enlarged as is more typical. Ultrasound can help depict discrete masses for targeted biopsy when skin-punch biopsy is negative. The palpable cords in the skin were caused by dermal lymphatics distended with tumor. (Courtesy of Wendie A. Berg, MD, PhD, FACR, Baltimore, MD. © Copyright 2006.)

The presence of echogenic calcifications within a sonographically and mammographically depicted mass can help affirm concordance (see Figs. 10, 31). When biopsying calcifications under ultrasound guidance, specimen radiography should be performed to assure calcification retrieval (Fig. 31) and use of larger, often vacuum-assisted devices helps assure adequate sampling.

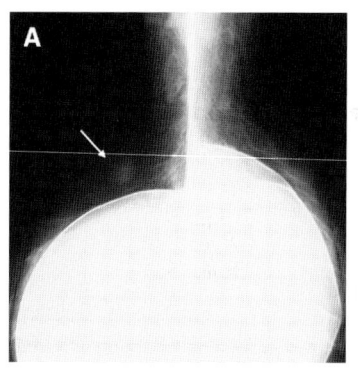

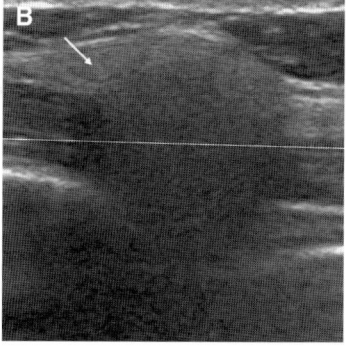

Fig. 34. Extracapsular silicone. This 56-year-old woman had silicone implants for 22 years and had them replaced by saline implants 6 years ago. (*A*) A mass was noted superior to the right implant on routine MLO mammograms (*arrow*), not visible on implant-displaced views. (*B*) Targeted ultrasound demonstrates "snowstorm" appearance of echogenic noise propagating deep to the mass (*arrow*), typical of a silicone granuloma or siliconoma, residual from prior extracapsular rupture of the original right silicone implant. (Courtesy of Wendie A. Berg, MD, PhD, FACR, Baltimore, MD. © Copyright 2006.)

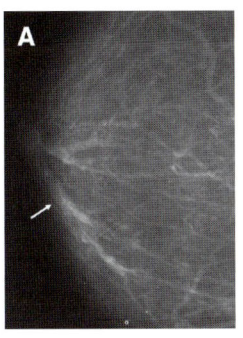

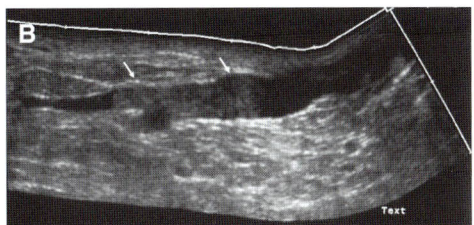

Fig. 35. A 50-year-old woman with spontaneous bloody nipple discharge. (*A*) Dilated duct (*arrow*) is noted behind the nipple on CC mammogram. (*B*) Extended-field-of-view ultrasound shows extensive intraductal mass (*arrows*). Excision confirmed benign papilloma. (Courtesy of Wendie A. Berg, MD, PhD, FACR, Baltimore, MD. © Copyright 2006.)

Inflammatory carcinoma

Ultrasound can contribute to the assessment of diffuse conditions such as suspected inflammatory carcinoma, often identifying one or more discrete masses (Fig. 33) as well as metastatic adenopathy [36,37]. Dilated lymphatics, diffuse increased echogenicity caused by edema, and skin thickening are evident on ultrasound of inflammatory carcinoma. Preferred diagnosis is by punch biopsy showing tumor in dermal lymphatics. When punch biopsy is nondiagnostic, however, ultrasound-guided biopsy of a discrete mass can help confirm the diagnosis.

Implants

Breast ultrasound has proven a to be helpful in evaluating the patient who has breast implants. At times the augmented breast has only a thin rim of overlying dense tissue that is suboptimally evaluated by routine and even implant-displaced mammographic views [38]; ultrasound can help improve

Table 1: Performance of combined mammography and breast ultrasound in symptomatic women

Study, Year [Reference Number]	Number of Cancers	Sensitivity (%)	Negative Predictive Value (%)	Patient Population/ Purpose of Study	Detection of Misses	Cancers Missed
Georgian-Smith, et al 2000 [51]	293	293 (100)	na	palpable, sensitivity of ultrasound to cancers	biopsy	none
Dennis, et al 2001 [52]	0	na	600/600 (100)	palpable, biopsy avoidance	biopsy or 2-year follow-up	none
Moy, et al 2002 [53]	6	0	227/233 (97.4)	palpable, determine NPV of combined ultrasound, mammography	tumor registry, 2-year follow-up	2 DCIS, 1 ILC, 3 IDC
Kaiser, et al 2002 [54]	6	6 (100)	117/117 (100)	thickening	biopsy or 14-mo follow-up	na
Shetty, et al 2002 [56]	0	na	186/186 (100)	palpable lump	biopsy or 2-year follow-up	na
Houssami, et al 2003 [55]	240	230[a] (95.8)	174/184 (94.6)	symptoms[a]	tumor registry, 2-year follow-up	na
Overall	545	529 (97.1)	1304/1320 (98.8)			

Abbreviations: DCIS, ductal carcinoma in situ; IDC, invasive ductal carcinoma; ILC, invasive lobular carcinoma; na, not applicable; NPV, negative predictive value.
[a] In the series of Houssami et al, 157 women who had cancer had a lump, and 114 who did not have cancer had a lump.
Adapted from Berg WA. Breast imaging. In: Chang AE, Ganz PA, Hayes DF, et al, editors. Oncology: an evidence-based approach. New York: Springer; 2006. p. 385.

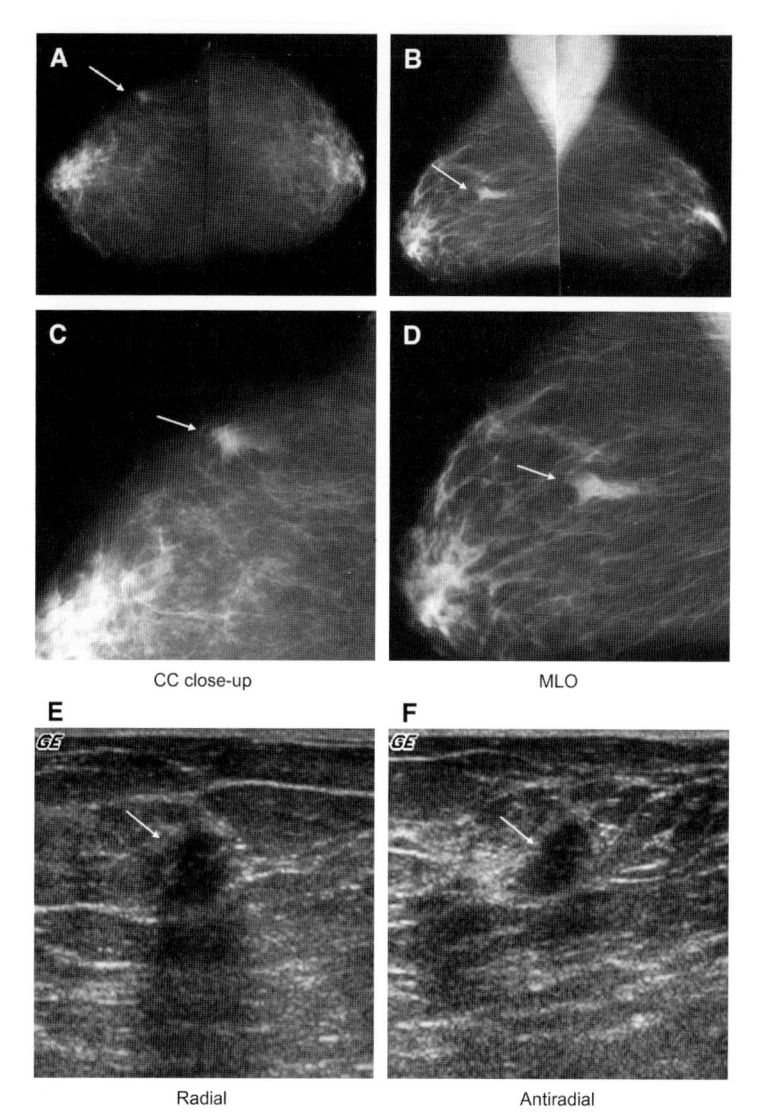

Fig. 36. Focal asymmetry was noted in upper outer right breast on screening (*A*) CC and (*B*) MLO mammograms (*arrows*) in this 60-year-old woman. The focal asymmetry (*arrows*) is seen better on photographic close-up (*C*) CC and (*D*) MLO mammograms. (*E*) Radial and (*F*) antiradial ultrasound performed at another facility showed a suspicious mass (*arrows*) thought to correspond to the mammographic asymmetry, and the patient was referred for biopsy. Repeat (*G*) radial and (*H*) antiradial ultrasound showed echogenic bands of tissue (*arrows*) compatible with normal variant. BBs were placed under ultrasound guidance, and the mammogram was repeated. (*I*) Spot-compression CC, (*J*) MLO, and (*K*) full mediolateral views confirm correspondence of the ultrasound-depicted finding (marked by the BBs placed at ultrasound) with the mammographic area of concern. This is a benign finding. (Courtesy of Wendie A. Berg, MD, PhD, FACR, Baltimore, MD. © Copyright 2006.)

cancer detection in this setting [39]. Although the cosmetic use of silicone implants has decreased dramatically since the Food and Drug Administration imposed restrictions on the use of silicone gel–filled implants for augmentation in 1992, women who have silicone implants continue to comprise a significant constituency within the population/age group now being screened. Ultrasound is useful in evaluating masses in women who have implants: extracapsular silicone with its snowstorm appearance (see Figs. 9, 34) [40] is readily distinguished from a suspicious mass needing biopsy. Ultrasound-guided biopsy can be performed safely in women who have implants, provided attention is given to maintaining a needle path parallel to the implant surface. Implant integrity, and particularly intracapsular rupture, is best evaluated with MR imaging [41,42].

Radial

Antiradial

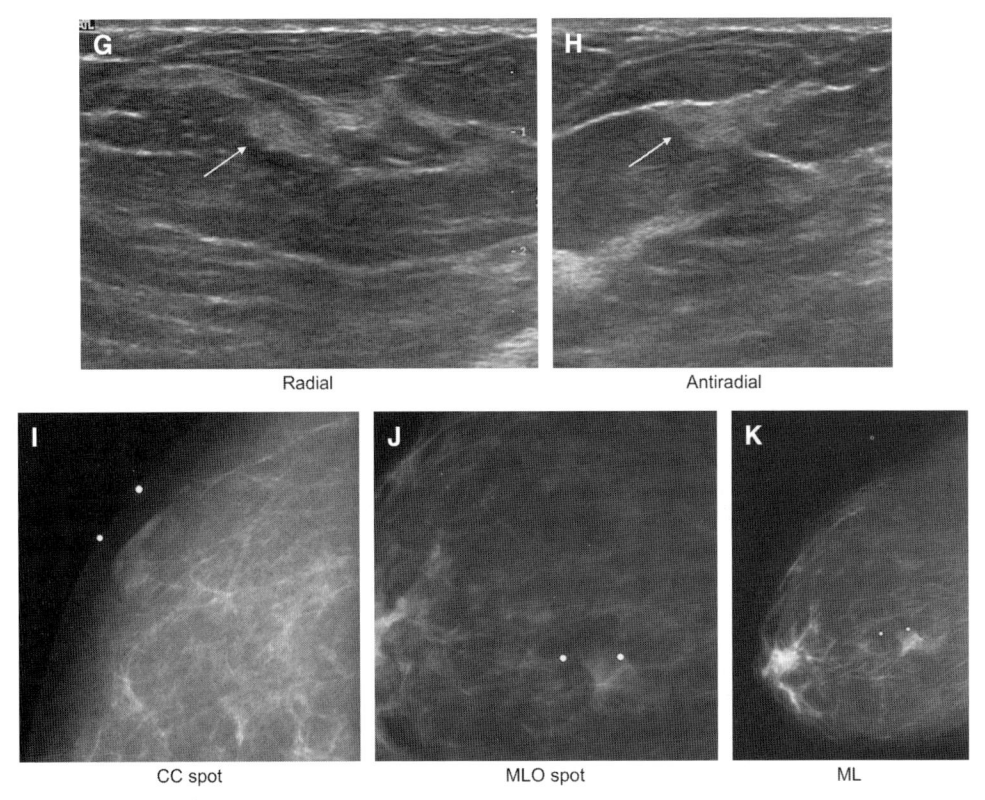

CC spot

MLO spot

ML

Fig. 36 (continued)

Nipple discharge

Any bloody nipple discharge warrants evaluation, as does spontaneous clear nipple discharge; the rate of malignancy with bloody discharge is as high as 13% [43]. Initial magnification CC and 90° lateral mammographic views can help exclude suspicious calcifications or subtle retroareolar masses. Ultrasound is an excellent adjunct to mammography in the evaluation of nipple discharge (Fig. 35). Initial clinical examination can help identify the likely orientation of the discharging duct based on the orientation of the discharging orifice within the nipple; sometimes a trigger point for the discharge can help direct attention to a particular location in the breast. Indeed, in one series ultrasound was superior to galactography, depicting 26 of 28 pathologic findings in ducts (93%), nine of which were missed at galactography [44].Ultrasound is far less painful and time-consuming than galactography as well, although, when there are multiple lesions, the full extent of intraductal masses may still be depicted better with galactography. MR imaging also is showing promise in evaluation of women who have nipple discharge [45].

Palpable abnormalities

Ultrasound is the initial test of choice in evaluating a palpable lump in a woman younger than 30 years of age [46]. Most palpable masses in such young women are caused by fibroadenomas [47]. The finding of a sonographically suspicious mass or a clinically suspicious mass without a sonographic correlate should prompt bilateral mammographic evaluation to define better the extent of malignancy, if any. At age 30 years and older, breast cancer is increasingly common, and mammography is the initial test of choice for symptomatic women.

At mammography, the palpable abnormality should be marked with a radiopaque marker. Tangential spot-compression views can help depict overlying skin thickening or retraction [48]. Magnification views are recommended to characterize the morphology, distribution, and extent of any associated suspicious calcifications; to help guide biopsy of the most suspicious areas [49]; and to characterize better the extent of any calcified DCIS component before treatment [50].

Strong evidence supports the use of ultrasound in addition to mammography in the evaluation of women who have a palpable mass or thickening

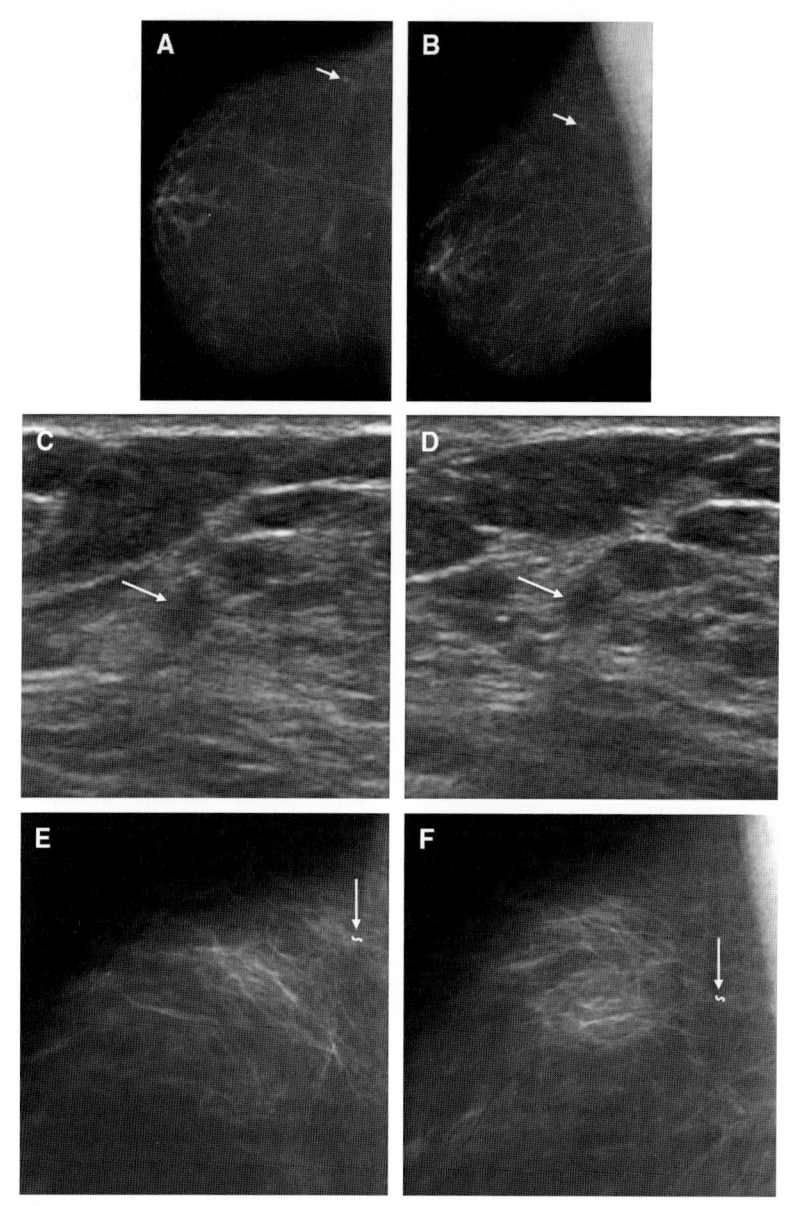

Fig. 37. (*A*) CC and (*B*) MLO mammograms demonstrate a 5-mm slowly enlarging mass in this 48-year-old woman who has history of contralateral cancer. Targeted (*C*) radial and (*D*) antiradial ultrasound demonstrated a subtle isoechoic irregular mass (*arrows*), thought to correspond to the mammographic abnormality. Ultrasound-guided core biopsy was performed with clip placement. Close-up (*E*) CC and (*F*) mediolateral mammograms immediately after ultrasound-guided biopsy show the clip in the expected location, confirming concordance of mammographic and ultrasound findings, with no residual mass. Histopathology of the core biopsy (and excision) showed granular cell tumor, concordant with the imaging findings. (*Courtesy of* Wendie A. Berg, MD, PhD, FACR, Baltimore, MD. © Copyright 2006.)

(Table 1) [51]. In the multi-institutional study of Georgian-Smith and colleagues [52], 616 palpable lesions were evaluated sonographically, and all 293 palpable cancers were depicted. Across several series in women who had symptoms (see Table 1), 529 of 545 cancers (97.1%) were depicted at ultrasound. A negative result after both mammography and ultrasound is highly predictive of a benign outcome, with a 98.8% negative predictive value across these series [52–57]. Nevertheless, final management of a clinically suspicious mass must be based on clinical grounds. When ultrasound is performed, the patient should direct the examiner to the area of concern, and the radiologist is best served by personally confirming the clinical findings and directly scanning over that area. At times, the area may be best appreciated with the patient seated or with the ipsilateral arm incompletely extended. By directly examining the area of clinical concern, the radiologist can determine the level of suspicion of the clinical finding and confirm concordance between the ultrasound and clinical findings. In the setting of mammographically fatty breasts and clinical findings consistent with normal variant fatty lobulation, ultrasound may not be necessary, provided the area of clinical concern is believed to have been included in the mammographic images.

Confirming concordance

For palpable abnormalities, direct correlation of the clinical findings with those on ultrasound is accomplished readily during scanning. Labeling of the ultrasound images should include the clock face, distance from nipple in centimeters (using the 38- or 50-mm transducer as a guide), transducer orientation, and any associated symptoms at that site (eg, "palpable," "nodularity," "tenderness," "area of pain").

To confirm correspondence of mammographic and ultrasound findings, a radiopaque marker can be placed over the ultrasound abnormality and the mammograms repeated (Fig. 36). This technique is successful for isolated superficial abnormalities but may be problematic when there are multiple findings or lesions deep in the breast. For suspicious subtle abnormalities, placement of a radiopaque marker at the biopsy site at the time of ultrasound-guided biopsy is strongly encouraged. A postbiopsy, postclip placement mammogram then can confirm concordance of the mammographic and the sonographic abnormalities (Fig. 37). Alternatively, a needle can be placed through the sonographic abnormality and the mammogram repeated before biopsy [58]. Cysts can be aspirated, and the mammogram repeated, if diagnostic uncertainty persists. Occasionally injection of air at the site of the biopsy can be used in a modern adaptation of the pneumocystogram. Air can be seen clearly as echogenic at ultrasound and persists for several hours at mammography, although current widespread use of ultrasound-deployable clips has largely replaced the injection of air. One clip, composed of carbon particulate, recently has been developed to be visible at follow-up ultrasound, although most clips are visible at follow-up ultrasound only when they are within a mass.

Summary

High-quality breast ultrasound after mammography is of great value in diagnostic breast imaging and is being explored for supplemental screening of selected groups of women [17]. This article provides a practical approach to mammographic-sonographic correlation. It reviews particular techniques that can help with this endeavor, including principles of correlating location, size, and lesion features and the use of anatomic landmarks. It reviews methods to confirm concordance, including the use of additional mammographic views, ultrasound-guided skin marker placement, and ultrasound-guided clip placement. Careful application of these techniques can help maximize the diagnostic performance of breast ultrasound. When ultrasound and mammography are properly correlated, abnormalities noted on screening mammography and even many palpable abnormalities can be dismissed as benign findings after complete work-up. For suspicious findings that can be seen sonographically, core biopsy under ultrasound guidance is a desirable and cost-effective alternative to stereotactic biopsy, MR imaging-guided biopsy, and surgical biopsy [59].

References

[1] D'Orsi CJ, Bassett LW, Berg WA, et al. Breast imaging reporting and data system BI-RADS: mammography. 4th edition. Reston (VA): American College of Radiology; 2003.

[2] Swann CA, Kopans DB, McCarthy KA, et al. Localization of occult breast lesions: practical solutions to problems of triangulation. Radiology 1987;163(2):577–9.

[3] Sickles EA. Practical solutions to common mammographic problems: tailoring the examination. AJR Am J Roentgenol 1988;151(1):31–9.

[4] Brenner RJ. Asymmetric densities of the breast: strategies for imaging evaluation. Semin Roentgenol 2001;36(3):201–16.

[5] Berg WA, Blume J, Cormack JB, et al. Operator dependence of physician-performed whole breast sonography: lesion detection and characterization. Radiology 2006;241(2):355–65.

[6] Memis A, Ozdemir N, Parildar M, et al. Mucinous (colloid) breast cancer: mammographic and US features with histologic correlation. Eur J Radiol 2000;35(1):39–43.

[7] Lam WW, Chu WC, Tse GM, et al. Sonographic appearance of mucinous carcinoma of the breast. AJR Am J Roentgenol 2004;182(4):1069–74.

[8] Berg WA, Gutierrez L, Ness-Aiver MS, et al. Diagnostic accuracy of mammography, clinical examination, US, and MR imaging in preoperative assessment of breast cancer. Radiology 2004;233(3):830–49.

[9] Tresserra F, Feu J, Grases PJ, et al. Assessment of breast cancer size: sonographic and pathologic correlation. J Clin Ultrasound 1999;27(9):485–91.

[10] Hilton SV, Leopold GR, Olson LK, et al. Real-time breast sonography: application in 300 consecutive patients. AJR Am J Roentgenol 1986; 147(3):479–86.

[11] Berg WA, Gilbreath PL. Multicentric and multifocal cancer: whole-breast US in preoperative evaluation. Radiology 2000;214(1):59–66.

[12] Moon WK, Noh DY, Im JG. Multifocal, multicentric, and contralateral breast cancers: bilateral whole-breast US in the preoperative evaluation of patients. Radiology 2002;224(2):569–76.

[13] Mendelson EB, Baum JK, Berg WA, et al. Breast imaging reporting and data system, BI-RADS: ultrasound. 1st edition. Reston (VA): American College of Radiology; 2003.

[14] Cawson JN. Can sonography be used to help differentiate between radial scars and breast cancers? Breast 2005;14(5):352–9.

[15] Brenner RJ, Jackman RJ, Parker SH, et al. Percutaneous core needle biopsy of radial scars of the breast: when is excision necessary? AJR Am J Roentgenol 2002;179(5):1179–84.

[16] Liberman L, Abramson AF, Squires FB, et al. The breast imaging reporting and data system: positive predictive value of mammographic features and final assessment categories. AJR Am J Roentgenol 1998;171(1):35–40.

[17] Berg WA. Supplemental screening sonography in dense breasts. Radiol Clin North Am 2004; 42(5):845–51 [vi].

[18] Leung JW, Sickles EA. Multiple bilateral masses detected on screening mammography: assessment of need for recall imaging. AJR Am J Roentgenol 2000;175(1):23–9.

[19] Esen G, Gurses B, Yilmaz MH, et al. Gray scale and power Doppler US in the preoperative evaluation of axillary metastases in breast cancer patients with no palpable lymph nodes. Eur Radiol 2005;15(6):1215–23.

[20] Sickles EA. Findings at mammographic screening on only one standard projection: outcomes analysis. Radiology 1998;208(2):471–5.

[21] Harvey JA, Fajardo LL, Innis CA. Previous mammograms in patients with impalpable breast carcinoma: retrospective vs blinded interpretation. 1993 ARRS President's Award. AJR Am J Roentgenol 1993;161(6):1167–72.

[22] Hussain HK, Ng YY, Wells CA, et al. The significance of new densities and microcalcification in the second round of breast screening. Clin Radiol 1999;54(4):243–7.

[23] Butler RS, Venta LA, Wiley EL, et al. Sonographic evaluation of infiltrating lobular carcinoma. AJR Am J Roentgenol 1999;172(2):325–30.

[24] Skaane P, Skjorten F. Ultrasonographic evaluation of invasive lobular carcinoma. Acta Radiol 1999;40(4):369–75.

[25] Rodenko GN, Harms SE, Pruneda JM, et al. MR imaging in the management before surgery of lobular carcinoma of the breast: correlation with pathology. AJR Am J Roentgenol 1996; 167(6):1415–9.

[26] Weinstein SP, Orel SG, Heller R, et al. MR imaging of the breast in patients with invasive lobular carcinoma. AJR Am J Roentgenol 2001;176(2): 399–406.

[27] Shetty MK, Watson AB. Sonographic evaluation of focal asymmetric density of the breast. Ultrasound Q 2002;18(2):115–21.

[28] Lee CH, Smith RC, Levine JA, et al. Clinical usefulness of MR imaging of the breast in the evaluation of the problematic mammogram. AJR Am J Roentgenol 1999;173(5):1323–9.

[29] Dershaw DD. Breast imaging and the conservative treatment of breast cancer. Radiol Clin North Am 2002;40(3):501–16.

[30] Yang WT, Tse GM. Sonographic, mammographic, and histopathologic correlation of symptomatic ductal carcinoma in situ. AJR Am J Roentgenol 2004;182(1):101–10.

[31] Moon WK, Myung JS, Lee YJ, et al. US of ductal carcinoma in situ. Radiographics 2002;22(2): 269–80 [discussion: 280–1].

[32] Fischer U, Kopka L, Grabbe E. Breast carcinoma: effect of preoperative contrast-enhanced MR imaging on the therapeutic approach. Radiology 1999;213(3):881–8.

[33] Hlawatsch A, Teifke A, Schmidt M, et al. Preoperative assessment of breast cancer: sonography versus MR imaging. AJR Am J Roentgenol 2002; 179(6):1493–501.

[34] Soo MS, Baker JA, Rosen EL. Sonographic detection and sonographically guided biopsy of breast microcalcifications. AJR Am J Roentgenol 2003; 180(4):941–8.

[35] Moon WK, Im JG, Koh YH, et al. US of mammographically detected clustered microcalcifications. Radiology 2000;217(3):849–54.

[36] Gunhan-Bilgen I, Ustun EE, Memis A. Inflammatory breast carcinoma: mammographic, ultrasonographic, clinical, and pathologic findings in 142 cases. Radiology 2002;223(3):829–38.

[37] Caumo F, Gaioni MB, Bonetti F, et al. Occult inflammatory breast cancer: review of clinical, mammographic, US and pathologic signs. Radiol Med (Torino) 2005;109(4):308–20.

[38] Egawa S, Matsumoto K, Iwamura M, et al. Impact of life expectancy and tumor doubling time on the clinical significance of prostate cancer in Japan. Jpn J Clin Oncol 1997;27(6):394–400.

[39] Hou MF, Ou-Yang F, Chuang CH, et al. Comparison between sonography and mammography for breast cancer diagnosis in oriental women after augmentation mammoplasty. Ann Plast Surg 2002;49(2):120–6.

[40] Harris KM, Ganott MA, Shestak KC, et al. Silicone implant rupture: detection with US. Radiology 1993;187(3):761–8.

[41] Everson LI, Parantainen H, Detlie T, et al. Diagnosis of breast implant rupture: imaging findings and relative efficacies of imaging techniques. AJR Am J Roentgenol 1994;163(1):57–60.

[42] Berg WA, Caskey CI, Hamper UM, et al. Single- and double- lumen silicone breast implant

integrity: prospective evaluation of MR and US criteria. Radiology 1995;197(1):45–52.

[43] Paterok EM, Rosenthal H, Sabel M. Nipple discharge and abnormal galactogram. Results of a long-term study (1964–1990). Eur J Obstet Gynecol Reprod Biol 1993;50(3):227–34.

[44] Hild F, Duda VF, Albert U, et al. Ductal orientated sonography improves the diagnosis of pathological nipple discharge of the female breast compared with galactography. Eur J Cancer Prev 1998;7(Suppl 1):S57–62.

[45] Orel SG, Dougherty CS, Reynolds C, et al. MR imaging in patients with nipple discharge: initial experience. Radiology 2000;216(1):248–54.

[46] Bassett LW. Imaging of breast masses. Radiol Clin North Am 2000;38(4):669–91 [vii–viii].

[47] Bartow SA, Pathak DR, Black WC, et al. Prevalence of benign, atypical, and malignant breast lesions in populations at different risk for breast cancer. A forensic autopsy study. Cancer 1987; 60(11):2751–60.

[48] Sickles EA. Combining spot-compression and other special views to maximize mammographic information. Radiology 1989;173(2):571.

[49] Morrow M, Schmidt R, Hassett C. Patient selection for breast conservation therapy with magnification mammography. Surgery 1995;118(4): 621–6.

[50] Holland R, Hendriks JH, Vebeek AL, et al. Extent, distribution, and mammographic/histological correlations of breast ductal carcinoma in situ. Lancet 1990;335(8688):519–22.

[51] Berg WA. Breast imaging. In: Chang AE, Ganz PA, Hayes DF, et al, editors. Oncology: an evidence-based approach. New York: Springer; 2006. p. 381–91.

[52] Georgian-Smith D, Taylor KJ, Madjar H, et al. Sonography of palpable breast cancer. J Clin Ultrasound 2000;28(5):211–6.

[53] Dennis MA, Parker SH, Klaus AJ, et al. Breast biopsy avoidance: the value of normal mammograms and normal sonograms in the setting of a palpable lump. Radiology 2001;219(1): 186–91.

[54] Moy L, Slanetz PJ, Moore R, et al. Specificity of mammography and US in the evaluation of a palpable abnormality: retrospective review. Radiology 2002;225(1):176–81.

[55] Kaiser JS, Helvie MA, Blacklaw RL, et al. Palpable breast thickening: role of mammography and US in cancer detection. Radiology 2002;223(3): 839–44.

[56] Houssami N, Irwig L, Simpson JM, et al. Sydney Breast Imaging Accuracy Study: comparative sensitivity and specificity of mammography and sonography in young women with symptoms. AJR Am J Roentgenol 2003;180(4): 935–40.

[57] Shetty MK, Shah YP. Prospective evaluation of the value of negative sonographic and mammographic findings in patients with palpable abnormalities of the breast. J Ultrasound Med 2002; 21(11):1211–6 [quiz: 1217–9].

[58] Kopans DB. Breast imaging. Philadelphia: Lippincott-Raven; 1998.

[59] Liberman L, Feng TL, Dershaw DD, et al. US-guided core breast biopsy: use and cost-effectiveness. Radiology 1998;208(3):717–23.

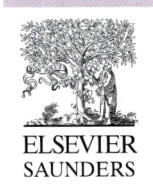

Breast Ultrasound MR Imaging Correlation

Basak Erguvan-Dogan, MD*, Gary J. Whitman, MD

- Targeted sonography for identification of MR imaging-detected breast lesions in patients who have a familial or a genetic predisposition to breast cancer
- Targeted sonography for identification of MR imaging-detected breast lesions in patients who have occult carcinoma of the breast
- Correlation of sonographic and MR imaging in other clinical settings
- Suggested protocol for management of lesions with suspicious enhancement on MR imaging
  Technique
  Clinical decision making
- Pitfalls
- Summary
- References

MR imaging of the breast has gained importance during the last decade because of its high sensitivity in detecting breast cancer. The most popular applications of breast MR imaging to date have been the following: searching for primary breast tumors in patients who have axillary metastases of unknown origin and negative findings on mammography and sonography; determining the extent of disease in breast cancer; monitoring response to neoadjuvant chemotherapy; screening patients who have a familial or a genetic predisposition to breast cancer; resolving cases of discordant imaging and clinical findings; and, less commonly, investigating the cause of nipple discharge in patients who have negative mammography, galactography, and sonography [1–9].

Despite the high sensitivity (94%–100%) of MR imaging in detecting invasive breast cancer, MR imaging has not been widely adopted as a screening or a diagnostic modality because of the wide range of specificity values (37%–97%) reported by various authors [3,10–12].

For lesions with suspicious or indeterminate enhancement features on MR imaging, further evaluation with percutaneous biopsy is necessary [13–15]. MR imaging–guided biopsy has several disadvantages, however: it is available only in selected centers, it is expensive, it requires trained personnel and scarce magnet time, it may not be tolerated by claustrophobic patients, and large patients may not be able to fit into the magnet. Unlike stereotactic breast biopsy followed by specimen radiography or real-time sonography-guided breast biopsy, MR imaging–guided biopsy does not allow confirmation of lesion sampling. It has been recommended that patients who have benign results on MR imaging–guided biopsy be referred for short-term follow-up MR imaging because sampling errors may occur.

As an alternative to MR imaging–guided biopsy for lesions with suspicious or indeterminate

---

Department of Diagnostic Radiology, Unit 57, The University of Texas M. D. Anderson Cancer Center, 1515 Holcombe Boulevard, Houston, TX 77030-4009, USA
* Corresponding author. Department of Diagnostic Radiology, Unit 1350, The University of Texas M. D. Anderson Cancer Center, P. O. Box 301439, Houston, Texas 77230-1439.
  E-mail address: basakerguvan@yahoo.com (B. Erguvan-Dogan).

enhancement features on MR imaging, various authors have used targeted sonography followed by ultrasound-guided biopsy [16–20]. This article reviews the literature to date on the use of targeted sonography for identification of MR imaging–detected breast lesions. Special attention is directed toward identification of MR imaging–detected breast lesions with targeted sonography in patients who have a familial or a genetic predisposition to breast cancer and targeted sonography for MR-detected lesions in occult carcinoma of the breast, two areas in which ultrasound following MR imaging seems to show great promise.

Targeted sonography for identification of MR imaging–detected breast lesions in patients who have a familial or a genetic predisposition to breast cancer

In women who have a genetically increased risk of breast cancer or a familial or a genetic predisposition to breast cancer, especially those who have *BRCA1* and *BRCA2* germline mutations, the lifetime risk of developing breast cancer may be as high as 80% [21]. For such women, breast cancer screening typically is initiated at a younger age than it is for other women. In young women, however, the density of the breast parenchyma may obscure lesions on mammography. Adjunctive modalities often are needed to enable detection of breast cancer at an early stage.

Clinical studies have shown that adding MR imaging to the screening regimen increases the sensitivity for the detection of breast cancer in high-risk women [22–25]. A multicenter trial by Lehman and colleagues [24] demonstrated that malignancies not suspected on mammography or sonography could be identified on MR imaging. Screening MR imaging yielded many false-positive findings, however, and resulted in twice as many unnecessary additional examinations and three times as many unnecessary biopsies as screening with mammography [24].

To the authors' knowledge, a study by Sim and colleagues [17] is the only study published to date investigating the use of targeted sonography to identify MR imaging–detected breast lesions in patients who have a family history of breast cancer. The investigators attempted to find sonographic correlates for 48 lesions that were categorized as category 4 and 5 according to the American College of Radiology's Breast Imaging Reporting and Data System (BI-RADS) on the basis of retrospective evaluation of MR imaging reports (Table 1) [26]. In most cases, sonography was performed as a directed examination to identify the MR imaging–detected lesion in question. The authors found sonographic correlates for 32 (67%) of the 48 lesions. Eleven (92%) of the 12 malignant lesions were visualized with sonography, whereas only 21 (58%) of the 36 benign lesions were seen with ultrasound. Breast cancer was present in 11 (34%) of 32 lesions with sonographic correlates and in 1 (6%) of 16 lesions without a sonographic correlate [17].

In the study by Sim and colleagues [17], 10 of the malignant lesions visualized on ultrasound were invasive tumors, and 2 were ductal carcinomas in situ (DCIS) [17]. The authors suggested that the higher rate of sonographic visualization of invasive cancers in their study (91%) than in a general population (58%) might be result from the smaller sample size [16,17]. The fact that the women included in the study by Sim and colleagues [17] were *BRCA1* and *BRCA2* mutation carriers and were more likely to have a higher prevalence of breast cancer than the general population may have resulted in a relatively higher percentage (25%) of malignant lesions than seen in the study by La Trenta and colleagues [16].

The study by Sim and colleagues [17] suggests that targeted sonography to identify MR imaging–detected breast lesions is a user-friendly, less time-consuming alternative to MR imaging–guided biopsy in women who have a familial or a genetic predisposition to breast cancer. Clinical studies with larger sample sizes are needed to determine whether follow-up or MR imaging–guided biopsy is the appropriate next step for management of MR imaging–detected lesions without sonographic correlates.

Targeted sonography for identification of MR imaging–detected breast lesions in patients who have occult carcinoma of the breast

MR imaging has a well-established role in the imaging work-up of women who present with metastatic adenocarcinoma in the axillary lymph nodes originating from an unknown primary tumor site. In this setting, the sensitivity of MR imaging has been reported to be 67% to 86% [8,9]. Demonstration of such tumors with targeted sonography may be problematic, however. First, in patients who have a history of contralateral breast cancer, the axillary metastases may be secondary to the contralateral malignant tumor. Second, lesions with enhancement on MR imaging may represent hormonal changes or nonspecific benign fibrocystic changes that may not be seen as discrete lesions on sonography.

To the authors' knowledge, only one study, by Obdeijn and colleagues [7], has been published to date on the use of combined targeted

Table 1: MR imaging–sonography correlation of breast lesions

Author (year) number of lesions	Study population	Total lesion correlation rate on ultrasound (%)	Malignant lesions correlated on ultrasound (%)	Benign lesions correlated on ultrasound (%)	False-negative rate for malignant lesions on ultrasound (%)
Obdeijn, et al (2000) N = 20	Axillary metastases in occult breast cancer	13/13 (100)	13/13 (100)	—	1/20 (MR imaging missed one cancer smaller than slice thickness)
LaTrenta, et al (2003) N = 93	General	21/93 (23)	9/19 (47)	12/74 (16)	10/19 (53)
Sim, et al (2005) N = 48	Familial risk of breast cancer	32/48 (67)	11/12 (92)	21/36 (58)	1/12 (8), (DCIS)
McMahon, et al (2005) N = 18	Axillary metastases in occult breast cancer	11/14 (79)	11/11 (100)	1/2 (50)	No false negatives; 2 false positives on MR imaging and ultrasound
Beran, et al (2005) N = 75	Documented or suspected breast cancer	65/73 (89)	Not stated[a]	Not stated[a]	Not stated[a]

Abbreviation: DCIS, ductal carcinoma in situ.
[a] The detection rates of benign and malignant lesions were not investigated separately by the authors. Therefore, an analysis similar to other studies cannot be made. Because the patients underwent breast MR imaging for documented or suspected breast cancer, presumably the majority of the lesions were visible by mammography or first-look sonography.

sonography and fine-needle aspiration in patients who had axillary metastases originating from an unknown primary tumor site (see Table 1). The authors performed breast MR imaging in 31 women who had axillary metastases and normal findings on mammography and clinical breast examination. MR imaging revealed a breast malignancy in 8 (40%) of the 20 patients who had no history of breast cancer, and MR imaging showed a second primary cancer in 3 (33%) of 11 patients who had a previous breast cancer. Two of the patients who had breast malignancies had two lesions each, so a total of 13 malignant breast lesions were identified on MR imaging. In 4 of the 20 patients who had no prior history of breast cancer, the axillary metastases originated from tumors at sites other than the breast; therefore, the success rate of MR imaging in detecting occult breast malignancies was 48% (13/27). Using sonography, the authors were able to identify all 13 lesions detected with MR imaging, and in all cases subsequent cytologic examination following fine-needle aspiration revealed malignancy [7].

In patients who have axillary metastases and no breast tumor identified on mammography and clinical examination, the radiologist's level of suspicion of breast cancer should be higher than it is for MR imaging–detected lesions with similar characteristics detected during screening of high-risk women. Even if the MR imaging appearance of a lesion suggests benignity, an attempt should be made to identify the lesion—or, in the case of multiple enhancing areas, the index lesion—on sonography.

The issue of first-look versus second-look breast sonography is important to consider. In most of the studies to date investigating the sensitivity of MR imaging in detecting occult carcinoma of the breast, only physical examination and mammography were performed before MR imaging; sonography was not performed [7–9]. In a recent study by McMahon and colleagues [20], however, both mammography and sonography were performed before MR imaging, and on targeted second-look sonography after MR imaging, the investigators were able to identify 78% of the breast tumors detected with MR imaging and missed on the initial sonograms (see Table 1).

In patients who had axillary metastases and no breast tumor identified on mammography and clinical examination, it may make sense to perform sonography before MR imaging. Sonography may reveal a mammographically and clinically occult malignant lesion and thus obviate the need for breast MR imaging. At The University of Texas M. D. Anderson Cancer Center, in patients who have axillary metastases and negative findings on clinical examination, bilateral mammography is followed by bilateral breast and axillary sonography and ultrasound-guided biopsy when necessary. If findings on sonography are negative, bilateral breast MR imaging is performed. If a lesion is identified on MR imaging, targeted sonography is performed, focusing on the specific location identified on MR imaging after three-plane reformatting to determine the exact distance of the lesion from the nipple and the skin. If a suspicious lesion is identified on MR imaging, and targeted sonography is negative, the patient is referred for MR imaging–guided percutaneous 9-gauge vacuum-assisted core biopsy.

Correlation of sonographic and MR imaging in other clinical settings

Sonographic correlation of lesions detected with MR imaging in various clinical settings seems to be less successful than for lesions detected at screening MR imaging in high-risk patients and those who

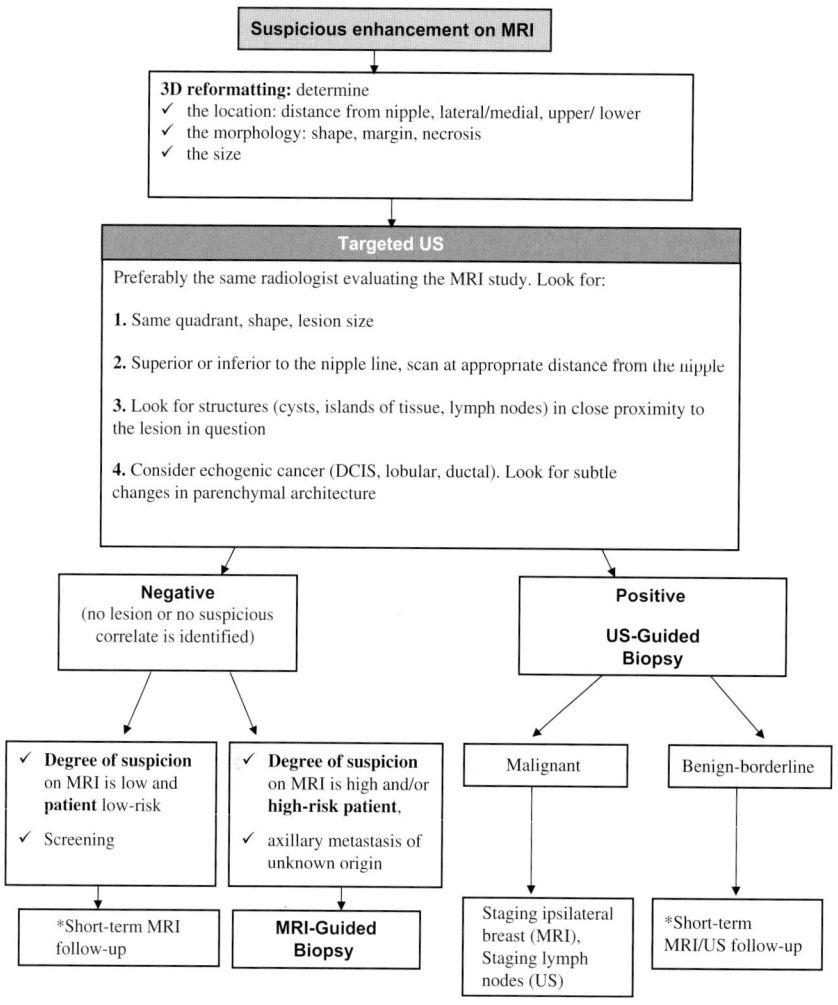

Fig. 1. Suggested management of breast lesions with suspicious enhancement on MR imaging (BI-RADS category 4 and 5 lesions). US, ultrasound. *, the patient, clinician, radiologist, and the pathologist should arrive at a consensus regarding management of these lesions. Short-term follow-up (BI-RADS category 3) or excisional biopsy may be considered.

have axillary metastases from an occult breast cancer. LaTrenta and colleagues [16] published a study of sonography for confirmation of 93 MR imaging–detected breast lesions (see Table 1). In that study, the authors found sonography correlates for only 21 (23%) of the 93 lesions identified on MR imaging. Furthermore, only 11 of those 21 lesions could be biopsied under ultrasound guidance; the remaining 10 lesions could not be confidently correlated with MR imaging findings. The reasons were listed as (1) uncertain correlation with the MR images (n = 3), (2) subtle nature of the sonographic finding (n = 2), (3) suspicion of a papillary lesion (n = 2), (4) recent result of an ipsilateral axillary node biopsy positive for breast carcinoma (n = 2), or (5) discretion of the surgeon (n = 1). The authors, however, were able to detect nearly 50% of the MR imaging–identified malignant lesions with targeted sonography. The uncertain indications for obtaining the MR imaging studies and the lack of standardized guidelines for interpreting benign and malignant lesions at the time of the study may have played a role in the rather large proportion of benign lesions (80%) referred for biopsy. Also, because sonographic correlation was poorer for benign lesions, almost half of all lesions were subjected to MR imaging–guided needle localization and surgical biopsy [16].

Results of a recent study by Beran and colleagues [19] were quite different (see Table 1). In that study, 191 women who had suspected or documented breast cancer underwent staging MR imaging. Fifty-two patients were found to have 73 additional lesions on MR imaging, 89% of which were identified on sonography. It is not clear what percentage of these lesions was malignant or how many malignant and benign lesions were identified by sonography. It is highly possible that one or more of the lesions identified on second-look sonography may have been visible on mammography or first-look sonography. It also is not clear what method of tissue sampling was used in this study. The high rate of correlation between sonography and MR imaging has been attributed mainly to both studies being performed by the same radiologist.

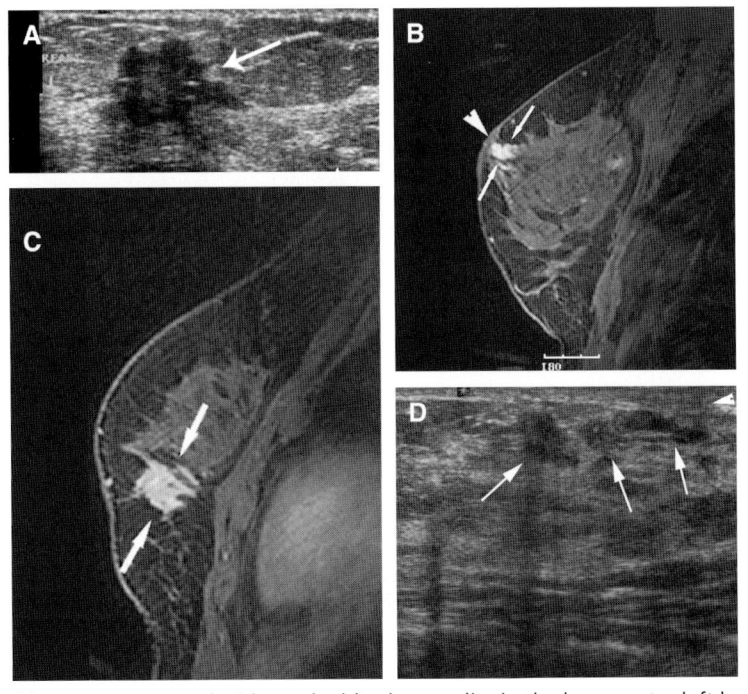

Fig. 2. A 51-year-old woman presented with a palpable abnormality in the lower outer left breast. Mammography revealed a suspicious mass in this region. (*A*) On sonography, a mass (*arrow*) was identified in the area of the palpable abnormality. Ultrasound-guided core biopsy revealed poorly differentiated invasive ductal carcinoma with DCIS. (*B*) MR imaging of the left breast revealed suspicious ductal enhancement (*arrows*) in the subareolar area (*arrowhead indicates nipple*). (*C*) MR imaging of the index mass (*arrows*) in the region of the palpable abnormality. (*D*) Second-look sonography revealed abnormal ductal structures (*arrows*) that resembled the MR imaging–detected abnormality in the subareolar region (*arrowhead indicates nipple*). Sonography-guided fine-needle aspiration revealed malignant cells. The patient underwent neoadjuvant chemotherapy and then mastectomy, which revealed multifocal cancer at 8 o'clock and in the subareolar area.

Suggested protocol for management of lesions with suspicious enhancement on MR imaging

In light of the available clinical data, the authors have developed a protocol for management of breast lesions with suspicious enhancement on MR imaging (BI-RADS category 4 or 5) that are detected by MR imaging alone (Fig. 1) [26].

Technique

If mammography and sonography were performed before MR imaging, knowledge of the findings on those studies may be helpful for determining the location of the lesion (Fig. 2). If the mammograms and the sonograms are interpreted as negative or are unavailable, it is important to perform three-plane reformatting and, when possible, to obtain maximum-intensity projection images of the fat-suppressed dynamic MR imaging data. The morphology and the dimensions of the MR imaging–detected lesion should be analyzed carefully.

When performing sonography to correlate with the MR imaging findings, the imager should be mindful of the differential diagnostic possibilities based on the MR imaging (for example, DCIS for non-masslike ductal enhancement, a fibroadenoma for a circumscribed mass with dark internal septations, and a lymph node for a mass bright on T2-weighted images with a fatty hilum). The distances from the nipple and the skin to the lesion, the quadrant or the clock-face location of the lesion, and any distinct cystic structures (such structures appear bright on T2-weighted images) close to the lesion and identifiable with sonography should be noted.

During targeted sonography, the distance from the nipple and the craniocaudal location with reference to the nipple are the most reliable data. Because the patient is positioned prone for MR imaging and supine for sonography, the lesion may project in different locations on each study. Also, slight compression applied to render the breast immobile during MR imaging may affect

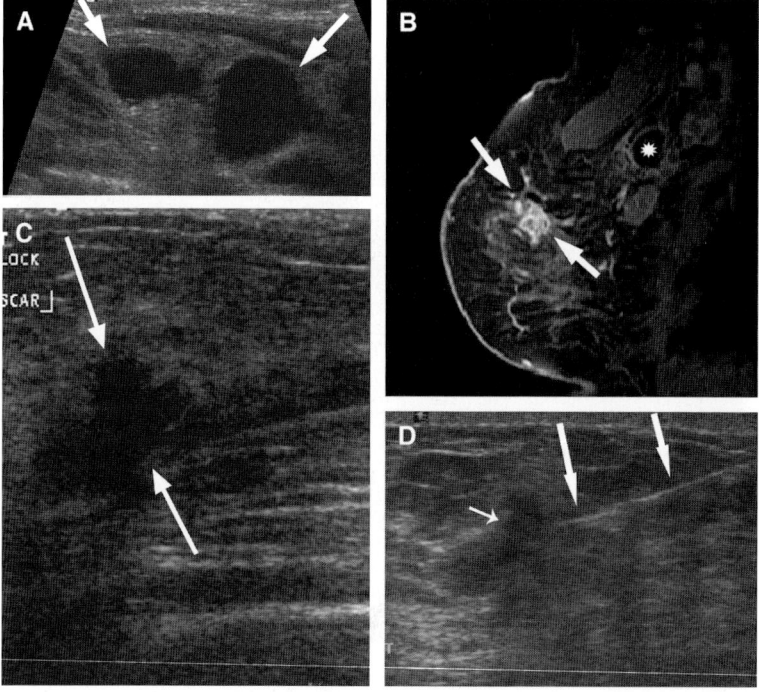

Fig. 3. A 52-year-old woman who had a history of DCIS in the right breast presented with palpable painless right axillary and supraclavicular lymph nodes 1 year after appropriate treatment (right-sided segmental mastectomy and radiation therapy). The patient underwent surgical biopsy of the right axillary lymph nodes that revealed metastatic adenocarcinoma. Findings on mammography and sonography were negative for a primary breast tumor. (*A*) Sonography showed metastatic axillary and supraclavicular lymph nodes (*arrows*). (*B*) Dynamic contrast-enhanced MR imaging revealed a 1.3-cm irregular mass lesion (*arrows*) with heterogeneous enhancement in the 10:00 to 11:00 region of the right breast, 4 cm from the seroma cavity (*asterisk*) on fat-suppressed three-dimensional fast spoiled gradient echo images. (*C*) Targeted sonography demonstrated a 1-cm hypoechoic lesion (*arrows*) separate from the seroma cavity. (*D*) Ultrasound-guided fine-needle aspiration (*large arrows point to the needle*) revealed poorly differentiated ductal carcinoma (*small arrow*).

the measurement of the distance from the lesion to the skin. It has been suggested that having sonography performed by the same radiologist who interpreted the MR imaging study may increase the sensitivity of targeted sonography [20]. At The University of Texas M. D. Anderson Cancer Center, the targeted post–MR imaging sonogram is performed by the same radiologist who interpreted the MR imaging, when possible.

Clinical decision making

When a lesion cannot be identified on targeted sonography, the indications for performing the MR imaging study in the first place and the lesion's degree of suspicion for breast cancer should be reviewed. Current data suggest that low-risk patients more commonly have benign lesions [23] and that benign lesions are significantly less likely to be visualized by targeted sonography [16–20]. Therefore, it may be safe to monitor closely low-risk patients who have no correlates identified on sonography. Lesions detected in patients who present with metastatic adenocarcinoma in the axillary lymph nodes originating from an unknown primary site (Fig. 3), lesions detected in women who have a familial or a genetic predisposition to breast cancer, and lesions with features highly suggestive of malignancy, such as thick peripheral rim enhancement, spiculated margins (Fig. 4), and irregular morphology, with or without early contrast washout, should be regarded with more suspicion and subjected to MR imaging–guided biopsy.

When sonography-guided biopsy reveals a borderline or a high-risk lesion, the clinician, the radiologist, and the pathologist should arrive at a consensus regarding management. When the management recommendations are unclear or controversial, excision should be considered, because the current understanding of the natural history of lesions initially discovered on MR imaging is limited.

Pitfalls

One of the challenges for radiologists performing breast sonography is confidently correlating the lesion visualized on sonography with the lesion visualized on MR imaging. A different solid lesion may be present at the site of an expected suspicious abnormality, or the original lesion detected by MR

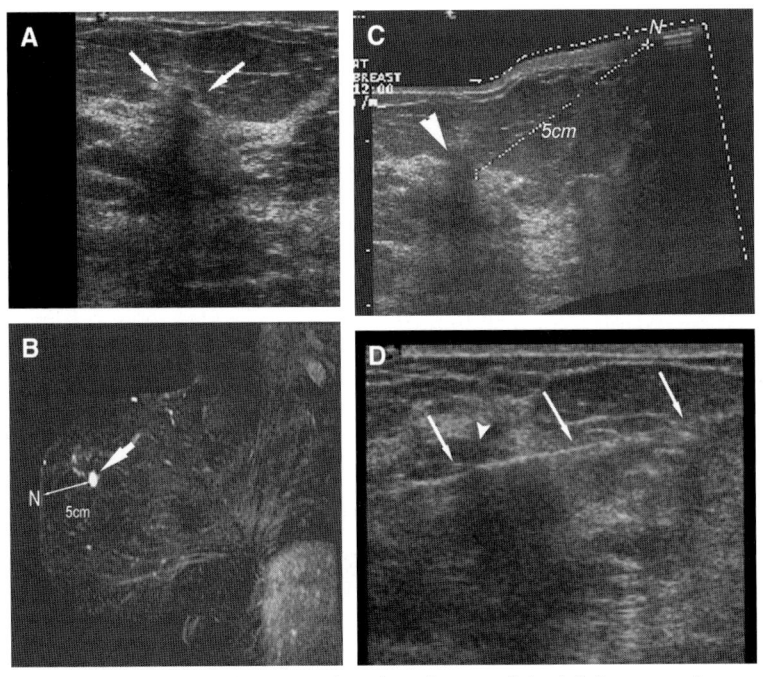

Fig. 4. A 57-year-old woman who had infiltrating ductal carcinoma of the left breast underwent bilateral breast sonography for staging. (*A*) On sonography, in addition to the known left breast carcinoma in the axillary tail region and metastatic left axillary lymphadenopathy, a subtle, 1-cm area of shadowing was noted in the 12:00 position of the left breast (*arrows*). (*B*) Bilateral breast MR imaging revealed a 1-cm oval mass with irregular borders (*arrow*) at 12:00 in the left breast. Note that the lesion, size, shape (taller than wide), and position (5 cm from the nipple [N] at 12:00) were similar on sonography and MR imaging. (*C*) Extended field of view sonography showed that the distance from the nipple (N) to the lesion (*arrowhead*) at 12:00 was 5 cm, identical to that on MR imaging. (*D*) Ultrasound-guided core biopsy (*arrows point to the needle*) revealed ductal hyperplasia without atypia and stromal fibrosis (*arrowhead*).

imaging may not be identified at all. The period between MR imaging and sonography should be kept to a minimum. Possible changes in the appearance of the breasts, influenced by weight and hormonal changes, should be noted. One option to aid with correlation is to use vitamin E capsules to mark the skin closest to the lesion visualized on MR imaging and to perform targeted sonography on the same day. Marking the skin with vitamin E capsules may be time-consuming, however, and it may be difficult to perform sonography on the same day as MR imaging.

Another method of confirming the identification of a targeted lesion is to place a clip marker after ultrasound-guided biopsy and to perform repeat dynamic MR imaging, especially if ultrasound-guided biopsy indicated that the lesion is benign. If the clip is not seen within the lesion in question on repeat dynamic MR imaging, MR imaging-guided biopsy may be warranted, depending on the clinical setting and the level of suspicion on MR imaging.

Summary

Sonographic correlation of breast lesions detected on MR imaging is becoming a popular alternative to MR imaging–guided interventions. Sonographic correlation allows ultrasound-guided biopsy and needle localization as well as sonographic follow-up. Clinical studies have shown that malignant lesions seem to be significantly more likely than benign lesions to have sonographic correlates. Success rates for correlation of sonography and MR imaging are higher in patients undergoing dynamic breast MR imaging for high-risk screening or to search for occult breast carcinoma that has metastasized to the axillary lymph nodes than in other patient groups.

Technically, it is important to perform three-plane reformatting to determine lesion characteristics such as size and morphology and to calculate the distance from the nipple and the skin. An appropriate differential diagnosis, based on the MR imaging findings, should be formulated. For lesions that are difficult to correlate, placing a vitamin E capsule or a marker on the skin may help with lesion localization. For lesions with discordant imaging and pathologic findings after targeted sonography and sonography-guided biopsy, placing a clip marker after biopsy and repeating the MR imaging may help to localize the lesion in question.

References

[1] Ishikawa T, Momiyama N, Hamaguchi Y, et al. Evaluation of dynamic studies of MR mammography for the diagnosis of intraductal lesions with nipple discharge. Breast Cancer 2004; 11(3):288–94.

[2] Daniel BL, Gardner RW, Birdwell RL, et al. Magnetic resonance imaging of intraductal papilloma of the breast. Magn Reson Imaging 2003; 21(8):887–92.

[3] Morris EA. Breast cancer imaging with MRI. Radiol Clin North Am 2002;40(3):443–66.

[4] Siegmann KC, Muller-Schimpfle M, Schick F, et al. MR imaging-detected breast lesions: histopathologic correlation of lesion characteristics and signal intensity data. AJR Am J Roentgenol 2002;178(6):1403–9.

[5] Morris EA. Cancer staging with breast MR imaging. Magn Reson Imaging Clin N Am 2001;9(2): 333–44.

[6] Orel SG, Dougherty CS, Reynolds C, et al. MR imaging in patients with nipple discharge: initial experience. Radiology 2000;216(1):248–54.

[7] Obdeijn IM, Brouwers-Kuyper EM, Tilanus-Linthorst MM, et al. MR imaging-guided sonography followed by fine-needle aspiration cytology in occult carcinoma of the breast. AJR Am J Roentgenol 2000;174(4):1079–84.

[8] Orel SG, Weinstein SP, Schnall MD, et al. Breast MR imaging in patients with axillary node metastases and unknown primary malignancy. Radiology 1999;212(2):543–9.

[9] Morris EA, Schwartz LH, Dershaw DD, et al. MR imaging of the breast in patients with occult primary breast carcinoma. Radiology 1997;205(2): 437–40.

[10] Gilles R, Guinebretiere JM, Lucidarme O, et al. Nonpalpable breast tumors: diagnosis with contrast-enhanced subtraction dynamic MR imaging. Radiology 1994;191(3):625–31.

[11] Heywang-Kobrunner SH. Contrast-enhanced magnetic resonance imaging of the breast. Invest Radiol 1994;29(1):94–104.

[12] Bone B, Aspelin P, Bronge L, et al. Sensitivity and specificity of MR mammography with histopathological correlation in 250 breasts. Acta Radiol 1996;37(2):208–13.

[13] Fischer U, Kopka L, Grabbe E. Magnetic resonance guided localization and biopsy of suspicious breast lesions. Top Magn Reson Imaging 1998;9(1):44–59.

[14] Liney GP, Tozer DJ, van Hulten HB, et al. Bilateral open breast coil and compatible intervention device. J Magn Reson Imaging 2000;12(6): 984–90.

[15] Helbich TH. Localization and biopsy of breast lesions by magnetic resonance imaging guidance. J Magn Reson Imaging 2001;13(6):903–11.

[16] LaTrenta LR, Menell JH, Morris EA, et al. Breast lesions detected with MR imaging: utility and histopathologic importance of identification with US. Radiology 2003;227(3):856–61.

[17] Sim LS, Hendriks JH, Bult P, et al. US correlation for MRI-detected breast lesions in women with familial risk of breast cancer. Clin Radiol 2005; 60(7):801–6.

[18] Ghai S, Muradali D, Bukhanov K, et al. Nonenhancing breast malignancies on MRI: sonographic and pathologic correlation. AJR Am J Roentgenol 2005;185(2):481–7.

[19] Beran L, Liang W, Nims T, et al. Correlation of targeted ultrasound with magnetic resonance imaging abnormalities of the breast. Am J Surg 2005;190(4):592–4.

[20] McMahon K, Medoro L, Kennedy D. Breast magnetic resonance imaging: an essential role in malignant axillary lymphadenopathy of unknown origin. Australas Radiol 2005;49(5):382–9.

[21] Ford D, Easton DF, Stratton M, et al. Genetic heterogeneity and penetrance analysis of the *BRCA1* and *BRCA2* genes in breast cancer families. Breast cancer linkage consortium. Am J Hum Genet 1998;62(3):676–89.

[22] Stoutjesdijk MJ, Boetes C, Jager GJ, et al. Magnetic resonance imaging and mammography in women with a hereditary risk of breast cancer. J Natl Cancer Inst 2001;93(14):1095–102.

[23] Kriege M, Brekelmans CT, Boetes C, et al. Efficacy of MRI and mammography for breast-cancer screening in women with a familial or genetic predisposition. N Engl J Med 2004;351(5): 427–37.

[24] Lehman CD, Blume JD, Weatherall P, et al. International Breast MRI Consortium Working Group. Screening women at high risk for breast cancer with mammography and magnetic resonance imaging. Cancer 2005;103(9):1898–905.

[25] Warner E, Plewes DB, Hill KA, et al. Surveillance of BRCA1 and BRCA2 mutation carriers with magnetic resonance imaging, ultrasound, mammography, and clinical breast examination. JAMA 2004;292(11):1317–25.

[26] American College of Radiology (ACR). ACR BI-RADS–magnetic resonance imaging. In: ACR breast imaging reporting and data system, breast imaging atlas. Reston (VA): American College of Radiology; 2003.

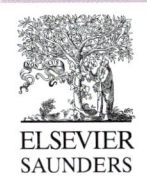

Ultrasound-Guided Breast Biopsies

Gary J. Whitman, MD[a,*], Basak Erguvan-Dogan, MD[a],
Wei Tse Yang, MD[a], Joella Wilson, BS[b], Parul Patel, MS[c],
Savitri Krishnamurthy, MD[d]

- Advantages of ultrasound-guided biopsies
- Disadvantages of ultrasound-guided biopsies
- Preprocedural preparations
- Ultrasound-guided core-needle biopsy
- Ultrasound-guided core biopsy of calcifications
- Ultrasound-guided vacuum-assisted core biopsy
- Ultrasound-guided fine-needle aspiration
- Ultrasound-guided marker placement
- Sonographic–pathologic correlation
- Summary
- Acknowledgments
- References

Currently, most breast biopsies are performed with percutaneous techniques; nearly all masses and some calcification clusters are biopsied with ultrasound guidance. In most breast imaging practices, ultrasound-guided breast biopsies are performed on a regular basis. In addition, sonography is commonly used to guide marker placements. This article reviews ultrasound-guided core-needle biopsy and fine-needle aspiration (FNA). The advantages and disadvantages of performing biopsies with sonographic guidance are discussed, and the techniques used in performing ultrasound-guided biopsies are reviewed. Sonographic–pathologic correlation is discussed.

Advantages of ultrasound-guided biopsies

Ultrasound-guided biopsies offer several benefits compared with mammographically guided, stereotactic, and surgical procedures. Ultrasound-guided procedures can be performed quickly, and they are less expensive than stereotactic and surgical procedures. Liberman and colleagues [1] noted that ultrasound-guided core biopsy decreased the cost of diagnosis by 56%, compared with the cost of surgical biopsy.

Sonography, unlike mammography and stereotactic biopsy units, does not use ionizing radiation. Furthermore, sonography provides access to all areas of the breast, independent of the breast size, as well as the regional (axillary, infraclavicular, supraclavicular, and internal mammary) and intramammary lymph nodes. In general, a lesion that can be visualized with sonography is accessible for an ultrasound-guided biopsy.

For ultrasound-guided biopsies, patients are positioned supine for medial lesions and in the

---

[a] Department of Diagnostic Radiology, The University of Texas M. D. Anderson Cancer Center, 1515 Holcombe Boulevard, Unit 1350, Houston, TX 77030, USA
[b] The University of Kansas School of Medicine, Mail Stop 1049, 3901 Rainbow Boulevard, Kansas City, KS 66160, USA
[c] State University of New York Upstate Medical University, 750 East Adams Street, Syracuse, NY 13210-2375, USA
[d] Department of Pathology, The University of Texas M. D. Anderson Cancer Center, 1515 Holcombe Boulevard, Unit 53, Houston, TX 77030, USA
* Corresponding author.
E-mail address: gwhitman@di.mdacc.tmc.edu (G.J. Whitman).

supine oblique position for lateral lesions. For example, if a right breast 10 o'clock mass is being targeted, the patient is positioned with a triangular foam wedge under the right shoulder (Fig. 1). This maneuver flattens the breast tissue. Thus there is less breast tissue for the needle to traverse, and the needle can be placed parallel to the skin surface and the transducer. Positioning for ultrasound-guided procedures is more comfortable for patients compared with mammographically guided procedures, in which the patient is seated, and stereotactic procedures, in which the patient is positioned prone.

One major advantage of sonography is that it allows for real-time monitoring of the targeted lesion and the needle. Real-time monitoring is particularly important in sampling firm lesions such as fibrotic fibroadenomas or movable lesions such as reactive axillary lymph nodes. Imaging in real-time allows the operator to see the needle in the lesion and to document the lesion moving with the needle motion during FNA. Real-time monitoring is particularly beneficial when FNA is performed on deep lesions with an oblique approach.

Disadvantages of ultrasound-guided biopsies

For targeting small groups of microcalcifications, stereotactic or mammographic guidance is preferred, because isolated calcifications and small clusters of calcifications are difficult to visualize on sonography. Regions of architectural distortion may present difficulties for targeting with sonography; in these cases mammographic, stereotactic, or perhaps MR imaging guidance may allow more precise targeting than ultrasound guidance. With mammography and stereotactic imaging, neighboring landmarks (ie, benign calcifications and intramammary lymph nodes) may be used to help to confirm the location of the targeted region. It usually is more difficult to identify these landmarks in a consistent location on ultrasound.

Preprocedural preparations

Before starting an ultrasound-guided biopsy, the procedure is explained to the patient and informed consent is obtained. The risks of bleeding and infection, which are low, should be discussed. The use of aspirin, nonsteroidal anti-inflammatory drugs, and anticoagulants increases the risk for bleeding. In the authors' practice, at the University of Texas, M. D. Anderson Cancer Center, the decision to proceed with a biopsy in a patient who has an elevated risk of bleeding is made by the breast imager performing the procedure and the patient. In general, ultrasound-guided core biopsies often are performed on patients taking aspirin and nonsteroidal anti-inflammatory agents but not on patients receiving anticoagulants. Ultrasound-guided FNAs often are performed on patients taking aspirin, nonsteroidal anti-inflammatory agents, and anticoagulants.

Before starting the procedure, the breast imager should scan the patient carefully and correlate the ultrasound findings with the findings on prior sonograms, mammograms, CT studies, and MR imaging studies. The patient then is positioned so that the operator can access the targeted lesion. The addition of a second, wall-mounted monitor can be particularly helpful so that the operator can approach the targeted lesion easily on either side of the patient (Fig. 2). The bed on which the patient lies should be on wheels so the operator can position the targeted area directly in line with the monitor. Also, the operator should be able to control the height of the bed so that he or she is in a comfortable position during the procedure. Some operators prefer to sit on a stool while performing ultrasound-guided procedures. Sitting can lessen the strain on the operator's lumbar spine

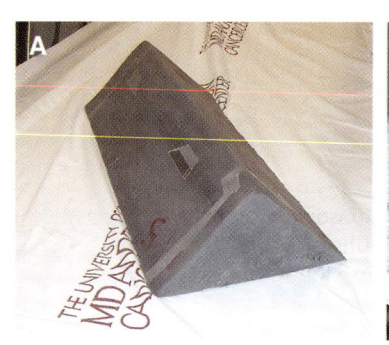

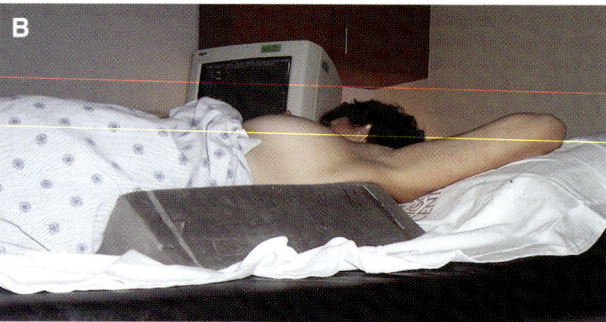

Fig. 1. (*A*) A triangular foam wedge used to help position the patient. (*B*) When a patient is positioned with the wedge under the left axillary region, the left lateral breast assumes a flatter configuration. Positioning in this manner facilitates placing the transducer parallel to the floor and the needle parallel to the transducer.

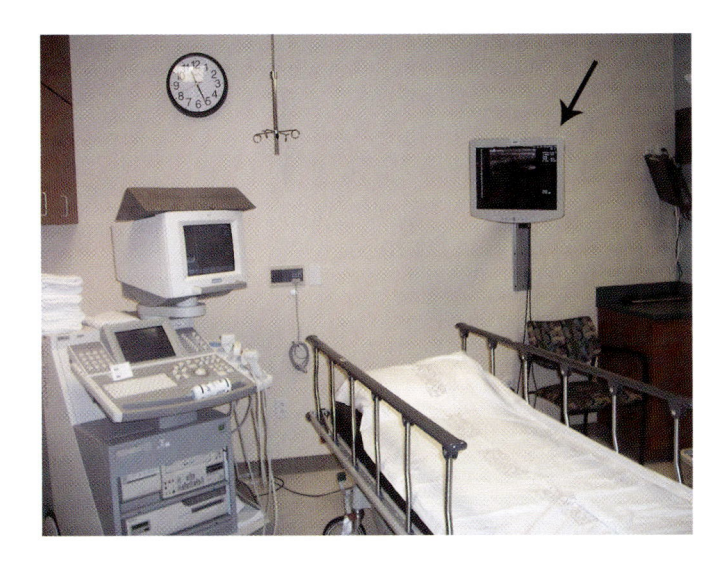

Fig. 2. It is helpful to have an extra wall-mounted monitor (*arrow*) so that an ultrasound-guided biopsy can be performed with the operator positioned on either side of the patient.

and help to facilitate a needle path parallel to the skin and the chest wall.

Before an ultrasound-guided biopsy is begun, the skin in the region of the targeted area is cleansed with povidone-iodine solution and alcohol. Alcohol facilitates transducer contact, so gel is not needed. The transducer also is soaked in alcohol and is placed directly on the skin over the targeted area.

For local anesthesia, lidocaine mixed with sodium bicarbonate (in a 1:10 lidocaine:sodium bicarbonate ratio) is injected subcutaneously. The sodium bicarbonate buffers the acidic bicarbonate and eliminates associated stinging. The lidocaine-bicarbonate solution must be used quickly; otherwise precipitation will occur. After the skin has been anesthetized, the lidocaine-bicarbonate solution is injected along the projected path of the needle and then around the lesion. The amount of local anesthetic may vary based on the location of the lesion, the breast composition, the type of procedure, and the number of needle passes. Usually 10 mL or less of local anesthetic is sufficient.

Ultrasound-guided core-needle biopsy

Ultrasound-guided core biopsies are the most frequently performed procedures in most breast ultrasound practices. Ultrasound-guided core biopsies may be performed with automated needles or vacuum-assisted biopsy devices. Most automated core biopsies are performed with 14-gauge needles, although 16-gauge and 18-gauge needles (Fig. 3) are used in many practices. The tissue yield is greater with a 14-gauge needle than with a 16-gauge (Fig. 4) or an 18-gauge needle, and in most breast imaging centers core biopsies are performed with 14-gauge long-throw (2.2-cm) automated needles. Parker and colleagues [2] noted that 14-gauge needles consistently provided intact cores for histopathologic analysis. Helbich and colleagues [3] compared the quantity and the quality of tissue harvested with 14-, 16-, and 18-gauge long-throw (2.2-cm) needles using stereotactic guidance. In that study the 14-gauge needles obtained significantly larger specimens, and the quality of the sample was significantly better with respect to tissue fragmentation, crush artifact, and adequacy of tissue for diagnosis than with the 16-gauge and the 18-gauge needles [3]. The investigators concluded that only 14-gauge needles should be recommended for breast biopsy [3].

When performing ultrasound-guided core biopsies, obtaining at least five scores is suggested, although some operators have achieved accurate results by routinely obtaining fewer cores. A long-throw (2.2-cm) needle is recommended. If the operator wishes to minimize the throw of the needle, short-throw (1-cm) needles may be used. The short-throw needles may be particularly helpful when the targeted lesion is located in the axilla, the axillary tail, near the chest wall, or near an implant.

In 1993, Parker and colleagues [4] first described ultrasound-guided automated core-needle biopsy. They reported a series of 181 breast lesions sampled with 14-gauge automated needles. Forty-nine lesions underwent subsequent surgical excision, with a correlation rate of 100% between the percutaneous biopsy results and the surgical biopsy results. Ultrasound-guided core biopsy revealed benign results in 132 lesions, and no cancers were identified in a follow-up period of 12 to 36 months. Since then ultrasound-guided core-needle biopsy has been shown to be cost-effective and accurate, and ultrasound-guided core biopsies have been performed extensively to sample nonpalpable breast lesions [4].

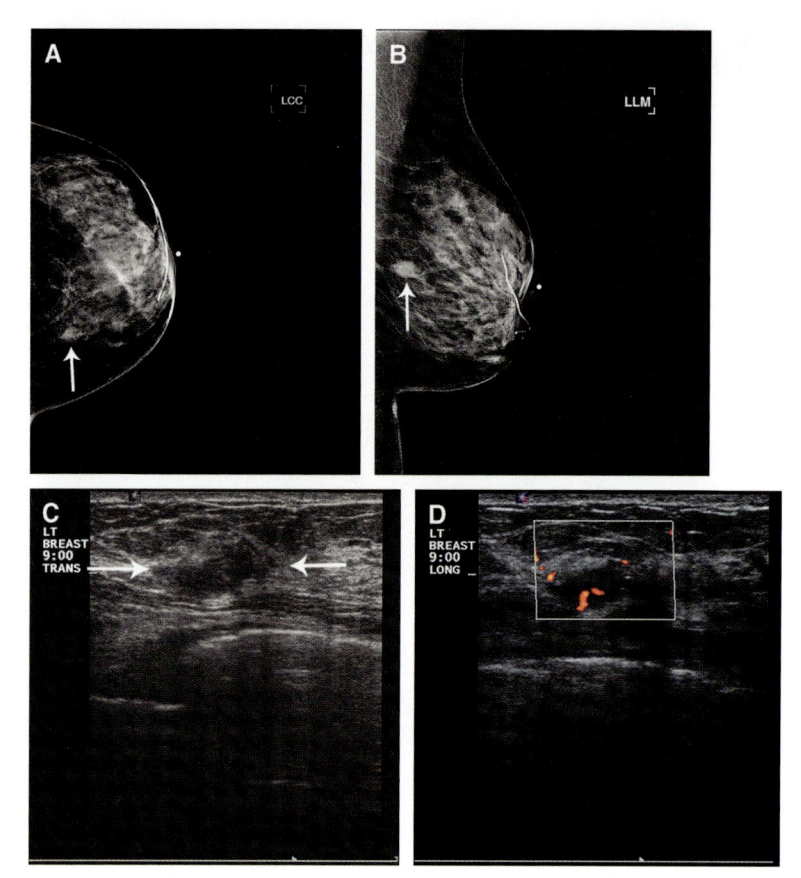

Fig. 3. A 65-year-old woman with invasive ductal carcinoma involving the left breast. (*A*) The left craniocaudal mammogram demonstrates an oval mass (*arrow*) in the medial left breast. (*B*) The left lateromedial mammogram shows the oval mass (*arrow*) in the posterior third of the breast. (*C*) Left breast transverse sonography shows a hypoechoic mass (*arrows*) with indistinct margins at 9 o'clock, corresponding with the mammographic findings. (*D*) Left breast longitudinal ultrasound with power Doppler imaging shows flow within the 9 o'clock mass. (*E*) Transverse left breast sonography shows the 18-gauge core biopsy needle (*black arrow*) at the edge of the 9 o'clock mass (*white arrow*). (*F*) Transverse left breast sonography demonstrates the 18-gauge core biopsy needle (*long arrow*) sampling the 9 o'clock mass (*short arrow*). (*G*) Longitudinal left breast ultrasound shows the 18-gauge needle (*short arrow*) within the 9 o'clock mass (*long arrow*). Pathology from the core-needle biopsy revealed invasive ductal carcinoma. Segmental resection revealed invasive ductal carcinoma and extensive DCIS extending close to the margins. The patient then underwent mastectomy that showed residual DCIS with no invasive carcinoma identified.

Crystal and colleagues [5] studied 715 consecutive ultrasound-guided core biopsies performed with a 14-gauge needle in 652 patients and found the sensitivity of sonographically guided core-needle biopsy for the diagnosis of breast cancer to be 96.3% with a false-negative rate of 3.7%. Thirty-one lesions (4% of all the cases) that were classified as benign on histopathology following ultrasound-guided core-needle biopsy underwent additional biopsy because of indeterminate pathologic findings (n = 5), disagreement between the imaging and the pathologic findings (n = 14), or patient or surgeon preference (n = 12). To evaluate these 31 lesions, 25 open excisional biopsies, 4 prone vacuum-assisted stereotactic biopsies, and 2 repeat ultrasound-guided core-needle biopsies were performed. Of the 31 lesions, 9 additional cancers were diagnosed. Five lesions were excised because of indeterminate pathologic findings; two were malignant, and three were benign (one radial scar, one intraductal papilloma, and one cellular fibroadenoma). Imaging–pathologic discordance led to repeat biopsy in 14 lesions, 7 of which were subsequently shown to be malignant. There were no malignancies in the 12 lesions excised because of the surgeon's or the patient's preference [5].

Crystal and colleagues [5] performed imaging follow-up (median, 39 months; range, 27–60 months) on 373 lesions with benign ultrasound-guided core-needle biopsy results. Mammographic

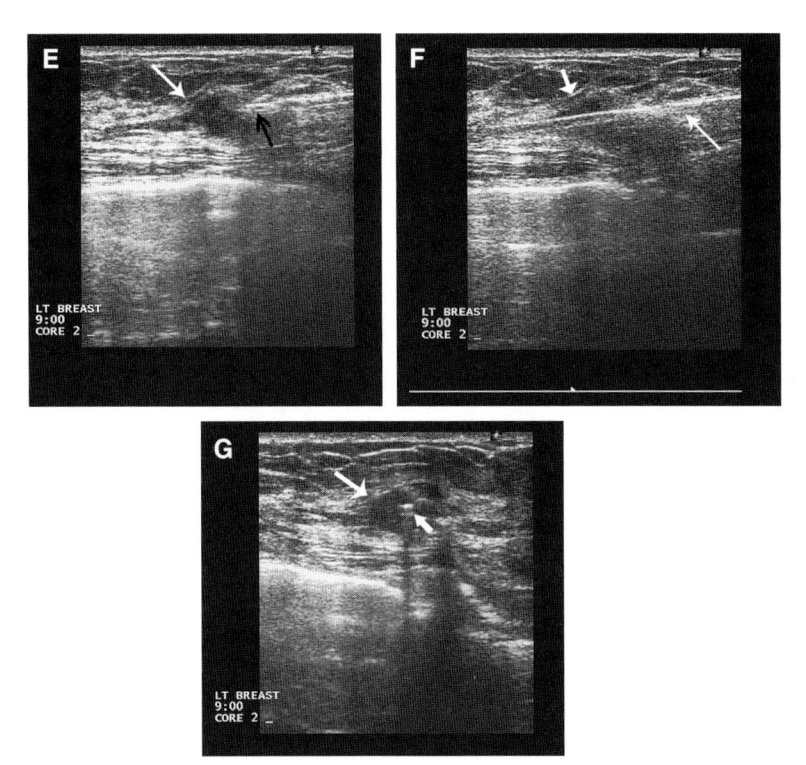

Fig. 3 (continued)

follow-up was recommended for women who had fatty breast parenchyma, and mammographic and sonographic follow-up was suggested for women who had dense breast tissue. During the follow-up period, three women presented with carcinomas at the site of a prior core-needle biopsy that had revealed benign results. The tumors ranged in size from 9 to 13 mm, and two of the three malignancies were invasive lobular carcinomas.

Dillon and colleagues [6] reviewed 2427 core-needle biopsies performed over a 5-year period. The authors reviewed 1279 ultrasound-guided core biopsies, 739 clinically guided core biopsies, and 409 stereotactic core biopsies. Malignancy was diagnosed in 1384 patients. Eighty-five patients were identified who had an initial benign core biopsy diagnosis followed by a diagnosis of cancer. The overall false-negative rate in the study was 6.1%; the false-negative rates for core biopsies performed with sonographic, clinical, and stereotactic guidance were 1.7%, 13%, and 8.9%, respectively.

Badoual and colleagues [7] performed a retrospective study on 110 consecutive malignant breast masses sampled with 14-, 16-, and 18-gauge automated core biopsy needles. Ultrasound-guided core-needle biopsies had a sensitivity of 100% for the diagnosis of breast cancer. When the ultrasound-guided biopsies were compared with surgical specimens, there was a 73.6% concordance for the assessment of tumor type. Most of the discrepancies were found in cases of invasive lobular carcinoma and mixed lobular and ductal carcinoma. In cases in which ductal carcinoma in situ (DCIS) was associated with invasive ductal carcinoma at surgery, ultrasound-guided core-needle biopsy revealed the DCIS component in 10% of cases. These findings probably result from the undersampling inherent in core biopsy techniques and the need for multiple cores, especially at the periphery of an invasive ductal carcinoma. In the study by Badoual and colleagues [7], the assessment of histologic grade of the core biopsy specimen and the surgical specimen was concordant in 73.1% of the cases. The concordance rates between core biopsy and excision for estrogen and progesterone receptors were 90.3% and 89.3%, respectively [7].

Ultrasound-guided core-needle biopsy is more accurate in larger (>1.5 cm) lesions than in smaller lesions (<1.5 cm) [8]. In addition, ultrasound-guided core biopsy requires a separate needle insertion before retrieval of each core, unless a coaxial technique is used, in which the needle is advanced through an introducer. Often, when multiple cores are obtained, the latter samples are composed predominantly of blood rather than the targeted tissue [9]. Also, for lesions with complex histopathology, core biopsy may provide incomplete characterization of the histopathologic findings [9].

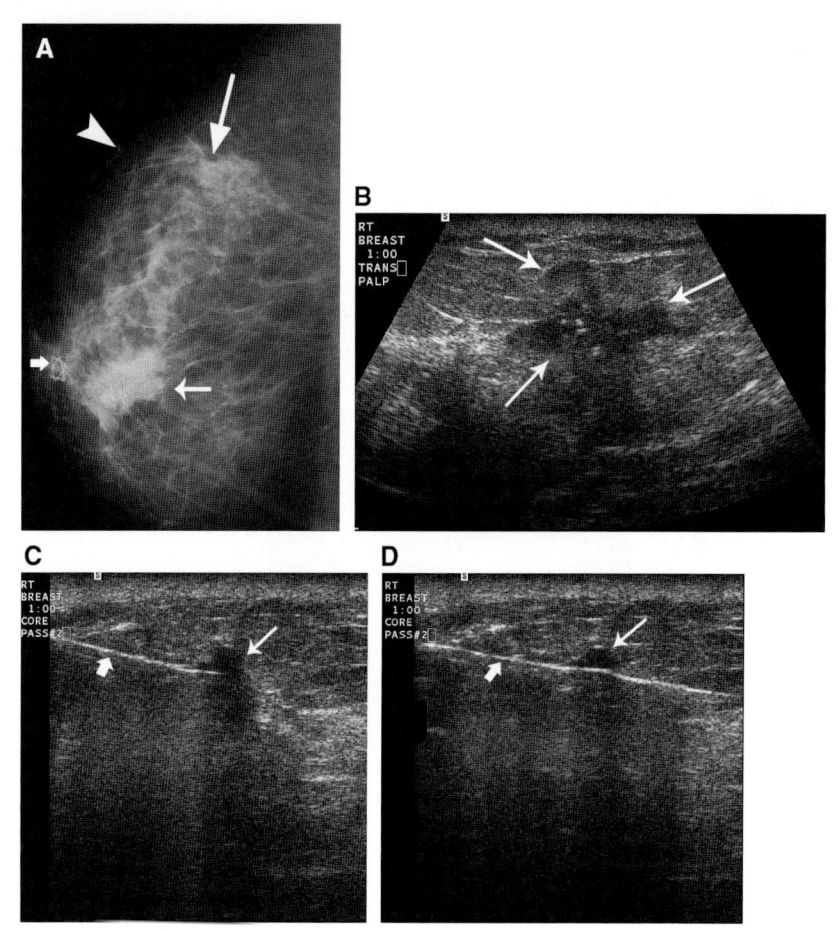

Fig. 4. A 52-year-old woman who presented with two palpable abnormalities in the right breast. Ultrasound-guided biopsies revealed multicentric carcinoma, with supraclavicular lymph node involvement. (*A*) The right craniocaudal mammogram demonstrates an irregular mass (*short thin arrow*) with spiculated margins and pleomorphic calcifications in the region of a palpable abnormality (palpable marker, *short thick arrow*) in the medial breast. An obscured mass (*long thin arrow*) is noted in the outer breast, in the region of a palpable abnormality (palpable marker, *arrowhead*). (*B*) Transverse right breast ultrasound at 1 o'clock shows an ill-defined, hypoechoic mass (*arrows*) with internal calcifications, corresponding to the mass seen in the medial breast on mammography. (*C*) Transverse right breast ultrasound shows the tip of a 16-gauge core biopsy needle (*short arrow*) within the targeted mass (*long arrow*) at 1 o'clock. (*D*) Transverse right breast ultrasound at 1 o'clock shows the 16-gauge needle (*short arrow*) sampling the hypoechoic mass (*long arrow*). (*E*) Longitudinal right breast sonography demonstrates the needle (*short arrow*) within the ill-defined mass (*long arrows*) at 1 o'clock. (*F*) Pathology from the core biopsy of the 1 o'clock mass demonstrates invasive ductal carcinoma with high-grade nuclear features. A group of tumor cells is noted with invasive edges (*arrows*) (hematoxylin and eosin, original magnification ×40). (*G*) Transverse right breast sonography demonstrates an ill-defined, hypoechoic mass (*arrows*) at 11 o'clock, corresponding to the obscured mass on the mammograms. (*H*) Transverse right breast ultrasound shows a FNA with a 21-gauge needle (*short arrow*) in the 11 o'clock mass (*long arrow*). (*I*) Cytology from the FNA of the right breast at 11 o'clock demonstrates clusters of ductal carcinoma cells (*long arrow*) and scattered, single ductal carcinoma cells (*short arrow*). The tumor cells have high nuclear grade features (Papanicalaou, original magnification ×40). (*J*) Longitudinal right supraclavicular ultrasound shows an oval, hypoechoic lymph node (*arrows*). (*K*) Transverse right supraclavicular ultrasound shows a FNA with a 21-gauge needle (*short arrow*) within the hypoechoic lymph node (*long arrow*). (*L*) Cytology from the right supraclavicular FNA demonstrates clusters of adenocarcinoma cells (*arrows*) in a background comprised of a pleomorphic population of lymphoid cells (Papanicalaou, original magnification ×20). The patient was treated with neoadjuvant chemotherapy before right mastectomy.

Ultrasound-Guided Breast Biopsies   609

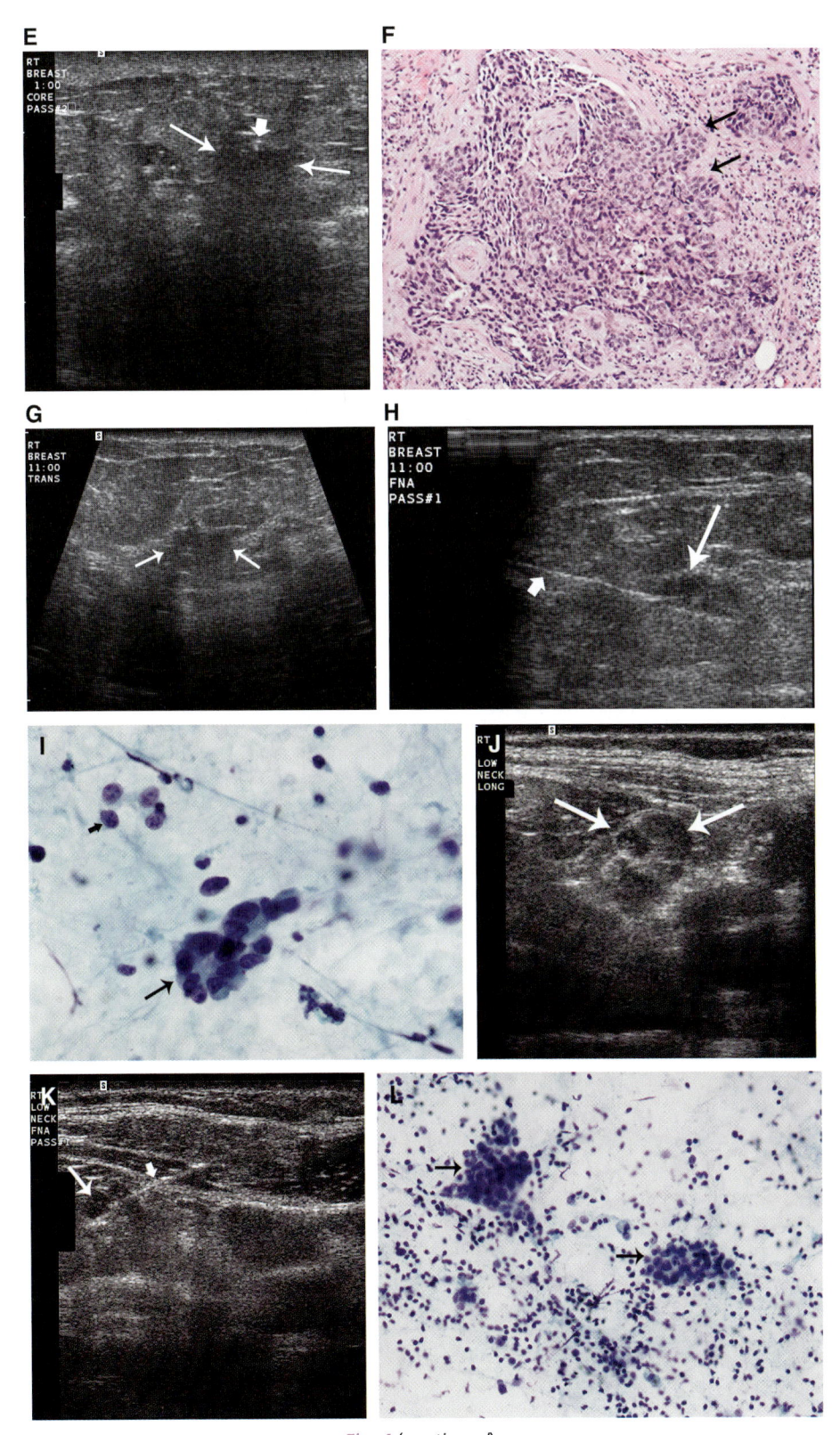

Fig. 4 (continued)

Ultrasound-guided core biopsy of calcifications

Although most ultrasound-guided core biopsies are performed on masses, core-needle biopsy may be used to sample calcifications within masses as well as calcifications without an associated mass. Ultrasound is less sensitive than mammography in demonstrating calcifications [10]. High-resolution transducers in the 10 to 13 MHz range, along with recent advances in ultrasound technology, have allowed the visualization of small echogenic spots without acoustic shadowing, corresponding to microcalcifications noted on mammography. Calcifications associated with malignant tumors are more likely to be seen on sonography than benign calcifications because most malignant calcifications are demonstrated within hypoechoic, malignant masses.

When calcifications are visualized with ultrasound, the calcifications are amenable to ultrasound-guided procedures, including core-needle biopsy [11,12]. Ultrasound-guided biopsy of calcifications may be pursued if the patient is unable to undergo stereotactic core biopsy for various reasons (eg, the patient's weight exceeding the weight limit for the stereotactic table, calcifications positioned very close to the nipple or the skin, or breast thickness less than 3 cm). When core-needle biopsy is performed, the calcifications are targeted as for a mass, and the needle should traverse the plane of the calcifications in two orthogonal views. After tissue acquisition, air along the biopsy track may obscure calcifications, making subsequent targeting difficult. When calcifications are targeted, post-biopsy specimen radiographs are useful to confirm the presence of calcifications. After core biopsy of calcifications, placement of a clip marker can be helpful to document appropriate sampling and to facilitate needle localization before excisional biopsy.

Ultrasound-guided vacuum-assisted core biopsy

Conventional core-needle biopsy techniques may be suboptimal for sampling calcifications, small (<1.5 cm) masses, and papillary lesions. Directional vacuum-assisted biopsy devices offer some advantages over automated core biopsy needles. Unlike automated core needles, directional vacuum-assisted biopsy probes do not require firing for tissue acquisition. Because of the vacuum, tissue can be acquired at a distance from the probe, not only in the line of fire. When vacuum-assisted probes are used with sonographic guidance, the probe usually is placed below the targeted lesion and then is raised toward the skin surface. Thus, the lesion is sampled from posterior to anterior. The vacuum-assisted probe may be inserted once, and multiple samples can be obtained following a single probe insertion. The samples obtained with 11- and 14-gauge vacuum-assisted devices are larger than those obtained with 14-gauge automated core needles. The larger size of the samples and the ability to obtain multiple cores with one probe insertion allow a substantially larger volume of tissue to be removed compared with a biopsy with a 14-gauge automated core needle [9].

Calcification retrieval is significantly improved with directional vacuum-assisted biopsy devices compared with automated core needles. Directional vacuum-assisted devices are more accurate than core needles in characterizing lesions containing atypical ductal hyperplasia (ADH), DCIS, and invasive carcinomas. Compared with core needles, directional vacuum-assisted instruments result in fewer ADH underestimates (percutaneous diagnosis of ADH for lesions containing DCIS) and fewer DCIS underestimates (percutaneous diagnosis of DCIS for lesions containing invasive ductal carcinoma) [9].

Parker and colleagues [8] performed 124 sonographically guided vacuum-assisted biopsies on masses less than or equal to 1.5 cm (mean size, 9.1 mm) in 113 patients. In this series there were 14 infiltrating ductal carcinomas, 1 infiltrating lobular carcinoma, 1 DCIS, 3 cases of ADH, 1 case of atypical lobular hyperplasia (ALH), and 1 phyllodes tumor. These were no underestimates of disease. The authors noted that vacuum-assisted biopsy reduced the possibility of a false-negative diagnosis because 90% of the time there was no remaining sonographic evidence of the targeted masses (which originally measured 1.5 cm in size or smaller). Thus, Parker and colleagues [8] concluded that one was less likely to miss a small mass (≤ 1.5 cm) with vacuum-assisted biopsy than with automated core-needle biopsy.

Percutaneous breast needle procedures may lead to displacement of benign or malignant epithelium into tissue away from the targeted lesion [13]. Epithelial displacement may occur in the breast parenchyma or in the skin. The displaced epithelial cells can lead to difficulties in histopathologic interpretation. Displaced DCIS may mimic infiltrating ductal carcinoma [9]. Parker and colleagues [8] noted that vacuum-assisted biopsies reduced the likelihood of epithelial displacement. Liberman [9] noted that firing automated core needles probably led to epithelial displacement. Thus, the reduced likelihood of epithelial displacement with vacuum-assisted devices is thought to result from the vacuum-assisted devices not being fired through the targeted tissue. In addition, larger volumes of tissue are acquired with vacuum-assisted biopsy devices than with automated core biopsies, and there is a greater likelihood of retrieving displaced epithelial cells. Also, the vacuum tends to pull the displaced epithelial cells into the probe rather than displace them [9].

Simon and colleagues [14] analyzed 71 11-gauge ultrasound-guided vacuum-assisted biopsies performed in 67 consecutive women. The vacuum-assisted biopsy findings were compared with excisional biopsy, mammographic follow-up and clinical follow-up findings (follow-up period, 1–19 months; mean, 9.2 months). Of the 71 lesions, 18 were malignant at vacuum-assisted biopsy. Vacuum-assisted biopsy revealed 1 case of ALH, 30 cases with specific benign diagnoses, and 22 cases with nonspecific benign diagnoses. In the case with a percutaneous biopsy diagnosis of ALH, excision revealed no evidence of atypia or malignancy. One benign finding was proven to represent carcinoma at excision. In this case, percutaneous vacuum-assisted biopsy revealed nonspecific benign findings. During the vacuum-assisted procedure, a hematoma developed that obscured the targeted lesion.

Simon and colleagues [14] noted that of the 71 vacuum-assisted biopsies, there was postprocedure bleeding lasting beyond 10 minutes in 5 of the cases (7%). In four of these cases, hemostasis was achieved with additional compression on the biopsy site of 20 minutes or less. In one case, 90 minutes of additional compression was required to achieve hemostasis. In one patient, a subcutaneous bleeding vessel required suturing at the time of percutaneous biopsy. The authors indicated that vacuum-assisted biopsy with sonographic guidance may be associated with a slightly higher risk of bleeding than vacuum-assisted biopsy with stereotactic guidance, probably because of the lack of breast compression during procedures performed with ultrasound guidance.

Ultrasound-guided fine-needle aspiration

In addition to ultrasound-guided core-needle biopsy and ultrasound-guided vacuum-assisted biopsy, ultrasound-guided FNA is an important technique. Although the Radiologic Diagnostic Oncology Group V reported that FNA of nonpalpable breast lesions was of limited value, successful FNA programs have been developed at centers with strong cytology support (Fig. 5) [15]. Ultrasound-guided FNA has been used at several centers to biopsy suspicious breast lesions (especially to document evidence of multifocal and multicentric disease) (see Fig. 4) and to biopsy suspicious regional lymph nodes (especially in the axillary region) (see Fig. 4). FNA is highly operator dependent; successful FNA programs require experienced, skilled operators performing the aspirations, proper slide preparation, and expert cytologic support. If an expert cytologist is on site at the time of the FNA, the adequacy of the sample can be determined, and a preliminary interpretation can be rendered before the patient is discharged from the breast imaging suite.

Although ultrasound-guided FNA is cheaper and quicker than ultrasound-guided core biopsy and ultrasound-guided vacuum-assisted biopsy, FNA has failed to gain universal acceptance in the United States. FNAs may result in insufficient samples, and core techniques provide more material with greater preservation of the architecture of the targeted lesion.

Boerner and colleagues [16] reviewed the cytologic findings from 1885 ultrasound-guided FNAs performed on 1639 patients. Cytologic specimens were correlated with pathology specimens in 851 cases and with clinical follow-up for a minimum of 2 years in 127 of the 274 patients who had benign solid lesions. Based on combined histologic and clinical follow-up, FNA had a sensitivity of 97.1% and a specificity of 99.1% (when definitive benign and malignant diagnoses were considered). The false-negative rate of 3.7% was attributed to sampling error and lesion characteristics. The false-positive rate of 0.68% was thought to result from interpretative error in assessing lesions with proliferative epithelium, such as fibroadenomas, radial scars, and epithelial hyperplasia. These investigators concluded that benign and inadequate FNA diagnoses should be correlated with the clinical and the imaging findings, and noncorrelative cases should undergo core-needle biopsy or excision.

Liao and colleagues [17] performed a retrospective study, evaluating 108 ultrasound-guided FNAs on sonographically suspicious, nonpalpable masses with a probabilistic reporting system. One hundred eight consecutive ultrasound-guided FNAs were diagnosed as positive (32), suspicious (8), atypical (11), benign (55), and unsatisfactory (2) when compared with 61 subsequent surgical specimens. Clinical and imaging follow-up was performed in the remaining 47 cases. All positive FNAs showed carcinoma on histology. The eight suspicious cases were shown to represent five carcinomas, two fibroadenomas, and one papillary lesion. Biopsy after atypical FNAs demonstrated four carcinomas, three fibroadenomas, and two papillary lesions. All 10 biopsies after benign FNAs showed fibrocystic changes. In two cases, the sonographic findings were suspicious, and FNA was unsatisfactory. In both these cases, histology demonstrated invasive lobular carcinoma [17].

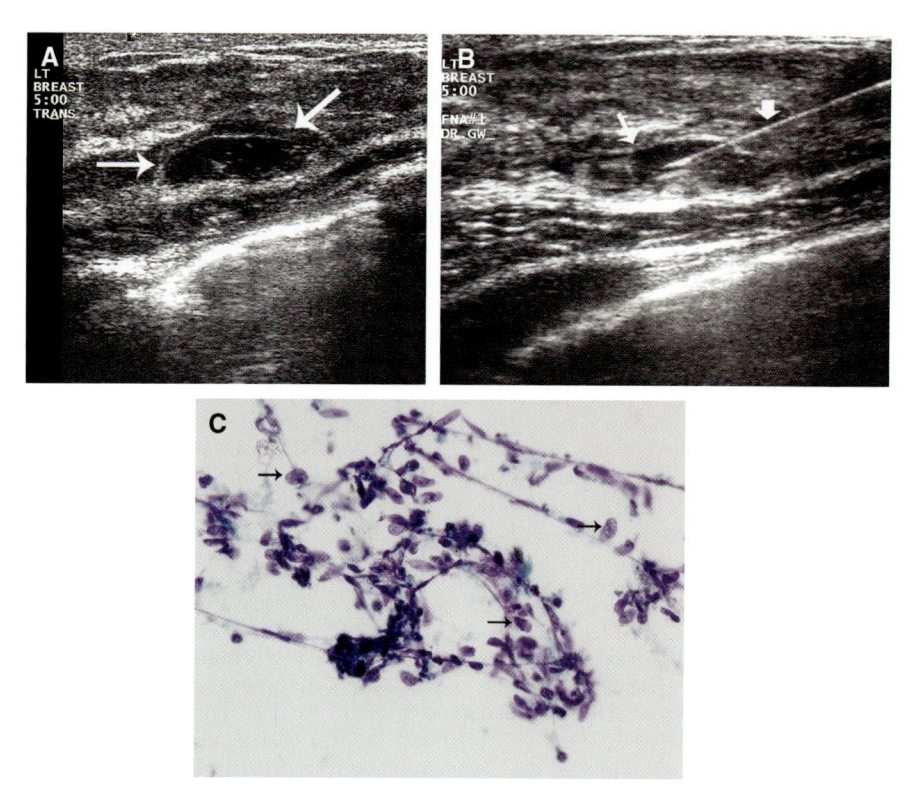

Fig. 5. Malignant spindle cell neoplasm in a 21-year-old woman diagnosed by FNA. (*A*) Transverse left breast sonography in the 5 o'clock region shows an oval, hypoechoic mass (*arrows*). (*B*) Transverse left breast ultrasound in the 5 o'clock region demonstrates a FNA with a 21-gauge needle (*short arrow*) within the hypoechoic mass (*long arrow*). (*C*) Cytology from the FNA of the left breast mass at 5 o'clock demonstrates malignant spindle cells (*arrows*) (Papanicalaou, original magnification ×40). The patient was treated with chemotherapy and radiation therapy before surgery.

In the study by Liao and colleagues [17], ultrasound-guided FNA was accurate in sampling nonpalpable masses. The positive predictive value (PPV) for FNA was 100% when the initial cytologic reading was positive. For suspicious FNAs, the PPV was 63%. For atypical FNAs, the PPV was 36%. The PPV for lesions classified as benign on FNA was 0%. At the University of Texas, M. D. Anderson Cancer Center, a FNA diagnosis of atypical, suspicious, or positive usually is followed immediately with an ultrasound-guided core-needle biopsy. Some masses such as papillary lesions (Fig. 6) and complex sclerosing lesions may require excisional biopsy for definitive diagnosis.

Ultrasound-guided marker placement

After an ultrasound-guided biopsy is performed, consideration should be given to placing a marker clip (Fig. 7) at the biopsy site with sonographic guidance. Placement of a marker clip is especially encouraged in cases with small (<1 cm) targeted lesions and in cases in which preoperative chemotherapy is likely to be administered [18]. Several types of marker clips have been described in which the clips are deployed through an introducing needle, allowing for a one-step, one-insertion technique [19–22]. The marker clips often are identifiable on sonography by their reflectivity, characteristic shape, and comet-tail artifact.

Immediately after a marker clip is placed with sonographic guidance, a two-view mammogram should be taken to document appropriate clip position. If the mammograms reveal that the marker clip is not in the desired location, the mammograms should be marked with a wax crayon to indicate the site of the biopsy. Clips may migrate because of hematomas, reabsorption of air at the biopsy cavity, or initial failure of the clip to attach to breast tissue [23].

Sonographic–pathologic correlation

After an ultrasound-guided biopsy, the operator must determine if the pathologic results are concordant with the imaging findings. The sonographic, mammographic, and MR imaging studies should be analyzed carefully, and the imager should

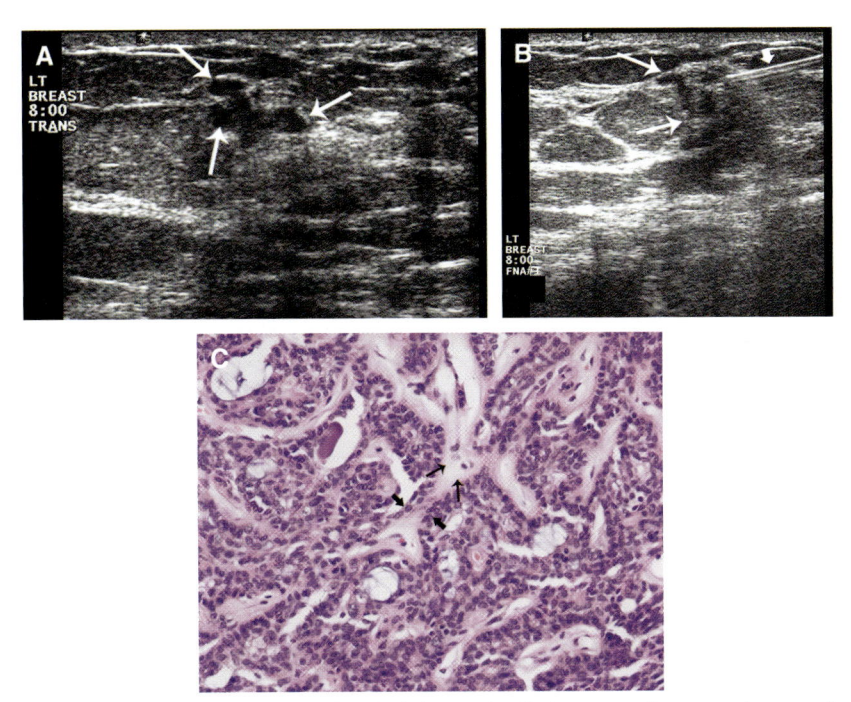

Fig. 6. A 59-year-old woman who presented with left nipple discharge underwent ultrasound-guided FNA, which revealed a papillary proliferative lesion. Subsequent excision demonstrated an intraductal papilloma. (A) Transverse left breast sonography in the 8 o'clock region shows an irregular ductal structure (*arrows*), with internal echoes. (B) Transverse left breast ultrasound shows a FNA of the irregular ductal structure at 8 o'clock (*long arrows*) with a 21-gauge needle (*short arrow*). Cytology revealed a papillary proliferative lesion, consistent with a sclerosing papilloma. (C) The patient underwent ultrasound-guided left breast needle localization and surgical excision. Pathology from the excision in the 8 o'clock region of the left breast demonstrates an intraductal papilloma with prominent fibrovascular cores (*long arrows*), surrounded by benign ductal epithelial cells (*short arrows*) (hematoxylin and eosin, original magnification ×40).

determine the likelihood of malignancy before the biopsy. In many practices, a ledger is used in which the operator writes down the imaging assessment before the biopsy (ie, likely malignant or category 4). When the pathology results are received, the operator should compare the histopathologic diagnosis with the imaging assessment before the biopsy. If the results are concordant, the operator should communicate the pathology findings to the patient and the referring physicians. In cases with concordant benign results, follow-up imaging usually is performed at 6 months or 1 year [24]. In cases with concordant malignant results or concordant potentially premalignant results (ie, ADH), the patient is referred for surgery or preoperative chemotherapy, depending on the stage of the recently diagnosed malignancy.

If the pathology results are discordant with the imaging findings, the operator should review the images, including the images from the biopsy procedure, and discuss the case with the pathologist [25]. Careful review of the biopsy procedure should be performed in an attempt to find a reason for the discordant results. Parikh and colleagues [26] identified four main causes of false-negative core biopsy results: (1) sampling the wrong lesion, (2) sampling a lesion with heterogeneous architecture, (3) suboptimal sampling (ie, patient movement or insufficient suction), and (4) procedural complications (ie, hematoma formation). After a discordant biopsy, repeat percutaneous biopsy or surgical excision should be performed [27].

Summary

Currently, in the United States, most initial biopsy procedures are performed with percutaneous techniques [28]. Most biopsies of masses are performed with sonographic guidance. Ultrasound-guided biopsies may be performed with vacuum-assisted probes, core needles, or fine needles. Percutaneous ultrasound-guided biopsies can provide a definitive histopathologic diagnosis and allow optimal surgical planning, which often results in a single surgical procedure with adequate margins [29]. Ultrasound-guided biopsy of benign conditions allows the avoidance of open biopsies for benign processes. In addition, ultrasound-guided biopsies are less

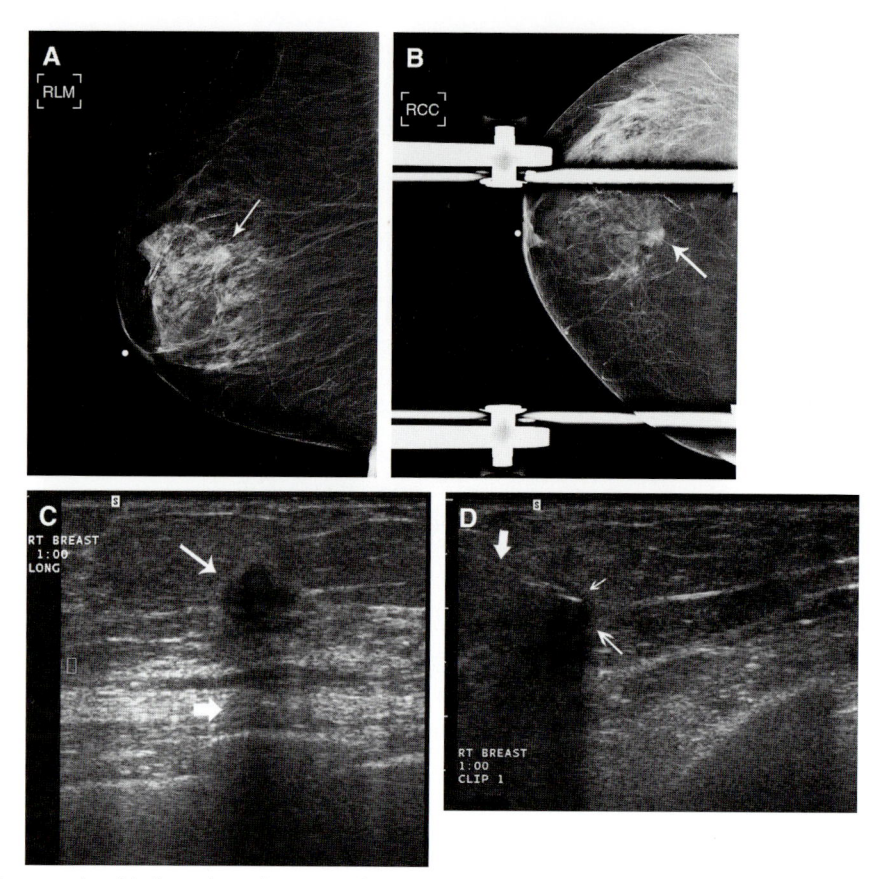

Fig. 7. Ultrasound-guided marker placement in a 79-year-old woman who had invasive ductal carcinoma. (*A*) Right lateromedial mammogram shows an irregular, spiculated mass (*arrow*) in the upper breast. (*B*) Right craniocaudal spot-compression mammogram demonstrates the irregular, spiculated mass (*arrow*) in the central breast, posterior to the nipple. (*C*) Transverse right breast sonography shows an irregular hypoechoic mass (*arrow*), corresponding to the mammographic findings. Ultrasound-guided core-needle biopsy was performed, revealing evidence of invasive ductal carcinoma. (*D*) Transverse right breast sonography in the 1 o'clock position shows an introducer (*thick arrow*) and a clip marker (Ultra CLIP II US, Inrad, Inc., Kentwood, MI, *small thin arrow*) in the superior portion of the known invasive ductal carcinoma (*long thin arrow*). Two weeks after clip placement, ultrasound-guided right breast needle localization was performed, followed by segmental mastectomy. Pathology showed invasive ductal carcinoma infiltrating adjacent adipose tissue. Right axillary sentinel lymph node biopsy showed no evidence of metastases.

invasive, less deforming, less expensive, and faster than surgical biopsies. Physicians who perform ultrasound-guided breast biopsies must use appropriate techniques and be willing to assume responsibility for establishing imaging–pathologic concordance and render appropriate referral and follow-up recommendations [24]. Ongoing developments in ultrasound equipment and tissue-acquisition devices will allow more breast biopsies to be performed more accurately in the future.

Acknowledgments

The authors thank Barbara Almarez Mahinda for assistance in manuscript preparation and Qiu Wu for photographic assistance.

References

[1] Liberman L, Feng TL, Dershaw DD, et al. US-guided core breast biopsy: use and cost-effectiveness. Radiology 1998;208(3):717–23.
[2] Parker SH, Lovin JD, Jobe WE, et al. Nonpalpable breast lesions: stereotactic automated large-core biopsies. Radiology 1991;180(2):403–7.
[3] Helbich TH, Rudas M, Haitel A, et al. Evaluation of needle size for breast biopsy: comparison of 14-, 16-, and 18-gauge biopsy needles. AJR Am J Roentgenol 1998;171(1):59–63.
[4] Parker SH, Jobe WE, Dennis MA, et al. US-guided automated large-core breast biopsy. Radiology 1993;187(2):507–11.
[5] Crystal P, Koretz M, Shcharynsky S, et al. Accuracy of sonographically guided 14-gauge core-needle

biopsy: results of 715 consecutive breast biopsies with at least two-year follow-up of benign lesions. J Clin Ultrasound 2005;33(2):47–52.

[6] Dillon MF, Hill AD, Quinn CM, et al. The accuracy of ultrasound, stereotactic, and clinical core biopsies in the diagnosis of breast cancer, with an analysis of false-negative cases. Ann Surg 2005;242(5):701–7.

[7] Badoual C, Maruani A, Ghorra C, et al. Pathological prognostic factors of invasive breast carcinoma in ultrasound-guided large core biopsies-correlation with subsequent surgical excisions. Breast 2005;14(1):22–7.

[8] Parker SH, Klaus AJ, McWey PJ, et al. Sonographically guided directional vacuum-assisted breast biopsy using a handheld device. AJR Am J Roentgenol 2001;177(2):405–8.

[9] Liberman L. Clinical management issues in percutaneous core breast biopsy. Radiol Clin North Am 2000;38(4):791–807.

[10] Hashimoto BE, Kramer DJ, Picozzi VJ. High detection rate of breast ductal carcinoma in situ calcifications on mammographically directed high-resolution sonography. J Ultrasound Med 2001;20(5):501–8.

[11] Teh WL, Wilson AR, Evans AJ, et al. Ultrasound guided core biopsy of suspicious mammographic calcifications using high frequency and power Doppler ultrasound. Clin Radiol 2000;55(5):390–4.

[12] Cleverley JR, Jackson AR, Bateman AC. Pre-operative localization of breast microcalcification using high-frequency ultrasound. Clin Radiol 1997;52(12):924–6.

[13] Liberman L, Vuolo M, Dershaw DD, et al. Epithelial displacement after stereotactic 11-gauge directional vacuum-assisted breast biopsy. AJR Am J Roentgenol 1999;172(3):677–81.

[14] Simon JR, Kalbhen CL, Cooper RA, et al. Accuracy and complication rates of US-guided vacuum-assisted core breast biopsy: initial results. Radiology 2000;215(3):694–7.

[15] Pisano ED, Fajardo LL, Caudry DJ, et al. Fine-needle aspiration biopsy of nonpalpable breast lesions in a multicenter clinical trial: results from the Radiologic Diagnostic Oncology Group V. Radiology 2001;219(3):785–92.

[16] Boerner S, Fornage BD, Singletary E, et al. Ultrasound-guided fine-needle aspiration (FNA) of nonpalpable breast lesions: a review of 1885 FNA cases using the National Cancer Institute-supported recommendations on the uniform approach to breast FNA. Cancer 1999;87(1):19–24.

[17] Liao J, Davey DD, Warren G, et al. Ultrasound-guided fine-needle aspiration biopsy remains a valid approach in the evaluation of nonpalpable breast lesions. Diagn Cytopathol 2004;30(5):325–31.

[18] Baron LF, Baron PL, Ackerman SJ, et al. Sonographically guided clip placement facilitates localization of breast cancer after neoadjuvant chemotherapy. AJR Am J Roentgenol 2000;174(2):539–40.

[19] Burbank F, Forcier N. Tissue marking clip for stereotactic breast biopsy: initial placement accuracy, long-term stability and usefulness as a guide for wire localization. Radiology 1997;205(2):407–15.

[20] Fajardo LL, Bird RE, Herman CR, et al. Placement of endovascular embolization microcoils to localize the site of breast lesions removed at stereotactic core biopsy. Radiology 1998;206(1):275–8.

[21] Phillips SW, Gabriel H, Comstock CE, et al. Sonographically guided metallic clip placement after core needle biopsy of the breast. AJR Am J Roentgenol 2000;175(5):1353–5.

[22] Guenin MA. Clip placement during sonographically guided large-core breast biopsy for mammographic-sonographic correlation. AJR Am J Roentgenol 2000;175(4):1053–5.

[23] Esserman LE, Cura MA, DaCosta D. Recognizing pitfalls in early and late migration of clip markers after imaging-guided directional vacuum-assisted biopsy. Radiographics 2004;24(1):147–56.

[24] Parker SH, Burbank F. A practical approach to minimally invasive breast biopsy. Radiology 1996;200(1):11–20.

[25] Nagi C, Jaffer S, Bleiweiss IJ. Mammographic-pathologic correlation in core biopsies of the breast. Semin Breast Dis 2005;8(3):138–43.

[26] Parikh J, Tickman R. Image-guided tissue sampling: where radiology meets pathology. Breast J 2005;11:403–9.

[27] Liberman L. Centennial dissertation. Percutaneous imaging-guided core breast biopsy: state of the art at the millennium. AJR Am J Roentgenol 2000;174(5):1191–9.

[28] Silverstein MJ, Lagios MD, Recht A, et al. Image-detected breast cancer: state of the art diagnosis and treatment. J Am Coll Surg 2005;201(4):586–97.

[29] Rogers LW. Breast biopsy: a pathologist's perspective on biopsy acquisition techniques and devices with mammographic-pathologic correlation. Semin Breast Dis 2005;8(3):127–37.

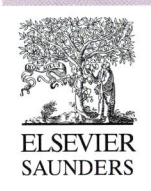

Cysts, Cystic Lesions, and Papillary Lesions

Gilda Cardenosa, MD[a,b,*]

- Simple cysts
- Oil cysts
- Other fluid collections
  Postoperative and traumatic fluid collections
  Galactoceles
- Abscesses
- Solitary papilloma
- Multiple peripheral papillomas
- Papillary carcinoma
- Complex cystic masses
- References

Simple cysts

Breast cysts are common. Although they are most often diagnosed in perimenopausal women and women in their 70s and 80s, cysts occur in women of all ages. Cysts that develop at the time of menopause usually decrease in size, and most such cysts resolve spontaneously unless the patient is treated with hormone replacement therapy. Clinically, patients who have cysts can present with one or several "lumps," focal tenderness, or, rarely, nipple discharge. When a cyst is inflamed, erythema may be present at the site of the "lump," and there may be associated tenderness. In many women, cysts are asymptomatic and are detected on screening mammography. A clinically detected breast mass cannot be characterized as a cyst on the basis of physical findings alone.

The mammographic appearance of cysts is variable. Cysts can occur as single or multiple, unilateral or bilateral masses of varying sizes and densities. Although many cysts are well circumscribed (Fig. 1A), some have obscured or ill-defined margins. Spiculation or distortion is rare. Calcifications can develop in the cyst wall or within cysts (referred to as "milk of calcium"). Unless associated with intracystic calcifications, most cysts are indistinguishable on mammography from other water-density masses, including malignancies, and thus sonography is indicated for further evaluation.

When appropriate criteria are applied to a lesion, breast ultrasound is 96% to 100% accurate in the diagnosis of cysts [1]. Sonographically, simple cysts are well-circumscribed, anechoic masses with sharp anterior and posterior walls, thin edge shadows, and posterior acoustic enhancement (Fig. 1B). During the real-time portion of the ultrasound study, the application of gentle pressure with the transducer directly over the cyst leads to elongation and compression if the cyst is not under tension. In some patients, slight movements or changes in the orientation of the transducer may be needed to demonstrate posterior acoustic enhancement, and in patients who have small (< 5 mm) or deep cysts, posterior acoustic enhancement may not be demonstrable. Reverberation artifacts may be present in the anterior wall of some cysts (Fig. 2). Less common appearances include the presence of echoes that are characterized by movement (eg, "gurgling") during the real-time portion of the study

---

[a] Virginia Commonwealth University, Richmond, VA, USA
[b] Department of Radiology, Virginia Commonwealth University Medical Center, Richmond, VA, USA
* Correspondence. Department of Radiology, Virginia Commonwealth University Medical Center, Box 980615, 1250 East Marshall Street, Richmond, VA 23298.
E-mail address: gcardenosa@vcu.edu

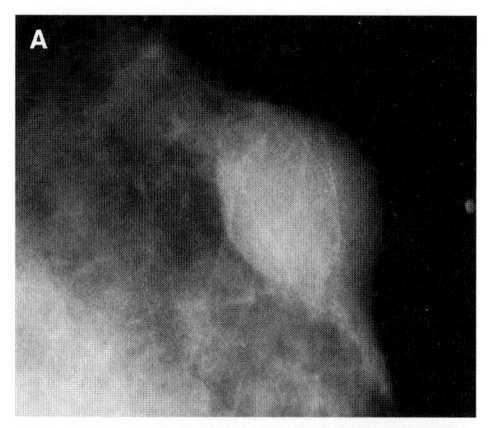

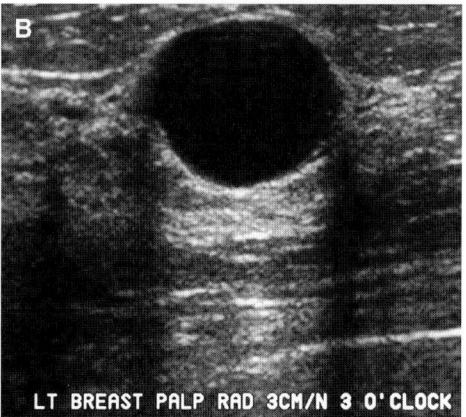

Fig. 1. Simple cyst. (*A*) Spot tangential mammographic view of a palpable mass in the left breast demonstrates a predominantly well-circumscribed mass corresponding to the site of clinical concern. (*B*) Ultrasound of the palpable mass in (*A*) in the radial projection shows a round, well-circumscribed, anechoic mass with posterior acoustic enhancement and thin edge shadows, diagnostic of a simple cyst.

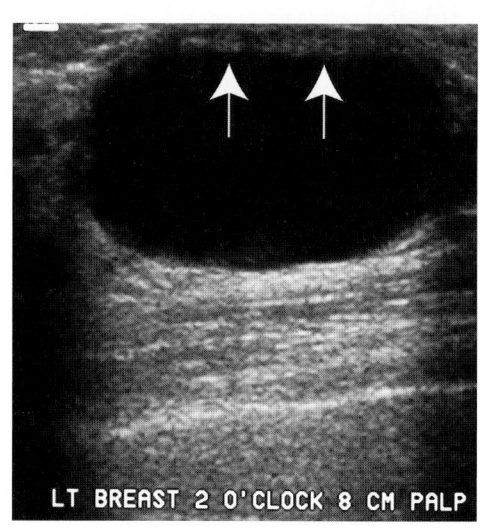

Fig. 2. Simple cyst. An oval, well-circumscribed, anechoic mass with posterior acoustic enhancement, diagnostic of a simple cyst. Echoes in the superficial aspect of the cyst (*arrows*) are consistent with reverberation artifact.

be seen. As these small cysts coalesce, the more characteristic appearance of the "single" cyst is seen. During real-time scanning, it is important to evaluate the entire lesion and to confirm that the septations are all thin. When the ultrasound findings are consistent with a simple cyst, the author

(Fig. 3) and persistent, nonmovable echoes that sometimes have an S-shaped interface (as in a ying-yang sign) with the more anechoic portion of the cyst (Fig. 4). In patients who have cysts associated with calcifications, high specular echoes may be seen in the cyst wall (mural calcifications) (Fig. 5) or within the cyst (intracystic calcifications).

In the early phases of cyst formation, as the acini making up the involved lobule begin to distend with fluid, tightly clustered, round, 1- to 2-mm anechoic areas are seen sonographically. These microcysts are separated by thin echogenic septations, and posterior acoustic enhancement may be present (Fig. 6). Although initially described as apocrine-lined cysts [2], histologically these areas are commonly a combination of small cystic spaces lined with either epithelial cells or cells characterized by apocrine metaplasia. As the acini continue to distend with fluid, clusters of small cysts may

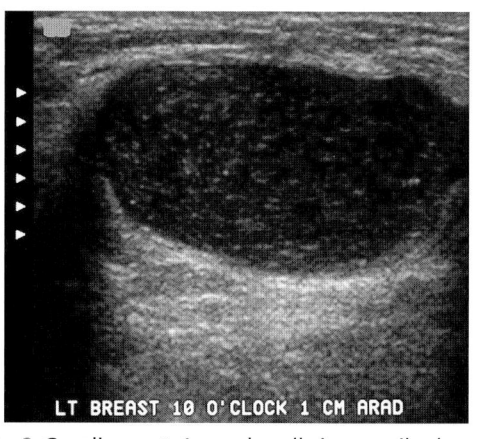

Fig. 3. Gurgling cyst. An oval, well-circumscribed mass with posterior acoustic enhancement and thin edge shadows as well as a myriad of internal specular echoes. If the transducer is held in a fixed position for a few minutes, these echoes are noted to move downward (as if falling) and to swirl, confirming that the mass is fluid filled. Unless the patient is symptomatic or requests aspiration, the author and colleagues do not routinely intervene when gurgling is noted during real-time scanning. The fluid aspirated from such cysts typically is serous and has no other distinguishing features.

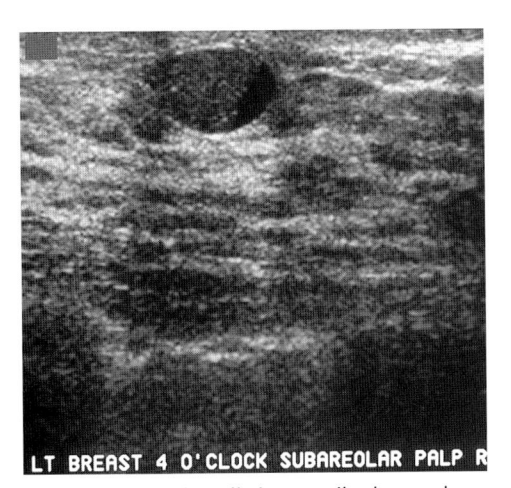

Fig. 4. Cyst. An oval, well-circumscribed, complex cystic mass characterized by an anechoic component having an abrupt linear interface with a more solid-appearing component. In patients who have complex cystic masses, aspiration is attempted; in most patients, fluid is obtained, the cyst collapses completely, and no residual abnormality is noted. If no fluid is obtained, a core needle biopsy is performed. The fluid aspirated from these cysts typically is serous and has no other distinguishing features.

and colleagues do not routinely recommend short-interval follow-up or core biopsy. If there is any question about the correct diagnosis, core biopsy is appropriate. If a core biopsy is undertaken, simple cysts decrease significantly in size and may disappear completely after the first or second pass through the lesion. Histologically, pieces of epithelial cell– and apocrine cell–lined cysts are reported after core biopsy of simple cysts.

The traditional approach to women presenting with a palpable mass has been palpation-guided aspiration. If no fluid is obtained, clinical follow-up, mammography, ultrasound, or excisional biopsy may be recommended. With the availability of modern ultrasound units, this traditional approach should be challenged for several reasons. First, cysts are benign and often multiple and do not need to be aspirated unless the patient experiences tenderness or there are atypical sonographic features. Some clinicians suggest that patients who have a palpable mass want the mass to go away. The author had found this not to be the case with most of her patients. What women want is the reassurance that what they feel is not breast cancer. If this reassurance can be provided with ultrasound (which offers the added benefit of evaluation of the tissue surrounding the palpable area), aspiration is not indicated, particularly because many cysts resolve spontaneously or fluctuate in size, and some recur within days of an aspiration. Second, failure to obtain fluid during palpation-guided aspiration does not mean that a lesion is not a cyst. When aspirations are done under ultrasound guidance, it is clear that some cysts are pushed away by the advancing needle and that, in other cases, a thickened wall is indented but not punctured by the needle (Fig. 7). The amount of compression that needs to be applied with the transducer to immobilize the mass so that it is not pushed ahead of the advancing needle and the amount of controlled pressure that needs to be exerted on the needle to allow it to puncture the cyst wall safely are best judged with sonographic guidance. Also, attempts to aspirate lesions may limit the value of subsequent mammographic and sonographic evaluations. Ideally, imaging studies should be done before any interventional procedures.

If the ultrasound criteria for a simple cyst are fulfilled, and the patient is asymptomatic, the author and colleagues do not recommend aspiration. They reassure patients that cysts are common, benign masses that fluctuate in size and tenderness with the menstrual cycle, may regress spontaneously, and often recur if aspirated. If the patient is symptomatic or if, because of atypical sonographic features, it is uncertain whether the finding is a cyst, the author and colleagues perform aspiration. They use ultrasound guidance for the aspiration to be sure that there is no residual abnormality after aspiration and because, in some cases, the needle may need to be redirected during the aspiration to ensure that all of the fluid is aspirated (eg, if the tip of the needle is against the cyst wall). For patients in whom there is concern about the presence of a mural or an intracystic abnormality, pneumocystography is performed: air is injected into the cyst cavity after the aspiration, and spot-compression magnification views of the mass are obtained to evaluate the cyst wall further. If there is adequate needle positioning (ie, the needle is in the center of the lesion) and no fluid is obtained, or if there is a residual abnormality after aspiration, core biopsies are done.

The author and colleagues routinely discard aspirated cyst fluid. Intracystic carcinomas are rare (accounting for 0.5% of all carcinomas and less than 0.1% of all cysts), and even when an intracystic carcinoma is present, findings on cytologic examination of the aspirated fluid are negative in more than half of the cases. They submit fluid for cytologic examination if they obtain bloody fluid after an atraumatic tap, if a patient has a residual abnormality after aspiration, if a patient requests the cytologic evaluation, or if a repeat aspiration is done in a patient who presents with rapid reaccumulation of fluid after initial aspiration. When a residual abnormality is seen after aspiration, in addition to

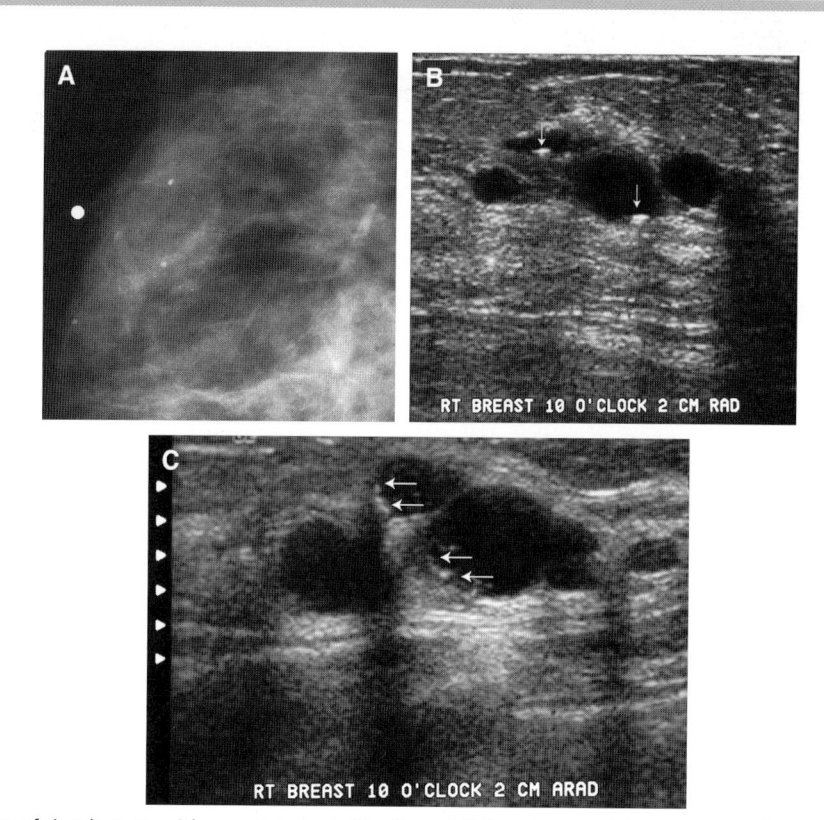

Fig. 5. Cluster of simple cysts with associated calcifications. (A) Spot tangential mammographic view of a palpable mass in the right breast demonstrates glandular tissue and some scattered round and punctate calcifications. (B) Ultrasound of the palpable mass in (A) in the radial projection demonstrates a cluster of four round and oval, well-circumscribed, anechoic masses, some with posterior acoustic enhancement, diagnostic of simple cysts. Echogenic calcifications (*arrows*) are noted. (C) Ultrasound of the palpable mass in (A) in the antiradial projection demonstrates three round, well-circumscribed anechoic masses, some with posterior acoustic enhancement, diagnostic of simple cysts. Calcifications (*arrows*) are identified.

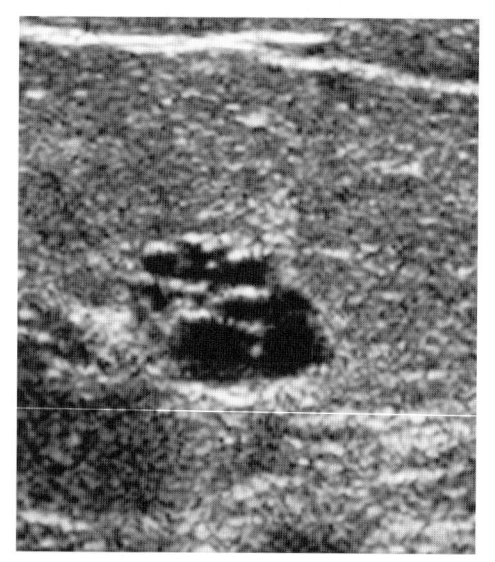

Fig. 6. Microcysts. Tightly clustered, round and oval, anechoic masses. The thin walls of the distending acini are noted as thin echogenic bands. Histologically, the cells lining these small cysts may be epithelial or demonstrate apocrine metaplasia.

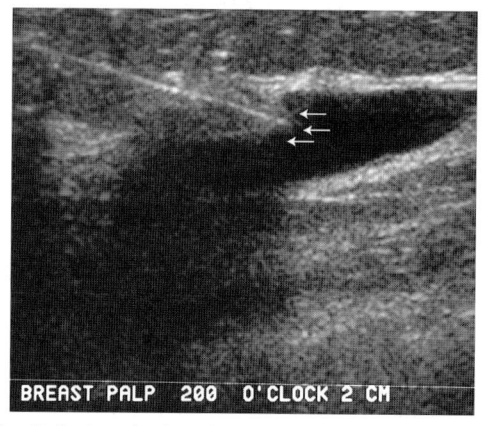

Fig. 7. Cyst aspiration. In some patients, during aspiration, the cyst wall is indented (*arrows*) but not penetrated by the advancing needle. The author and colleagues prefer to use ultrasound guidance for all cyst aspirations because sonography enables them to judge how much compression to apply to keep the mass from moving ahead of the advancing needle and how much pressure to exert on the needle to ensure that it punctures the wall of the mass.

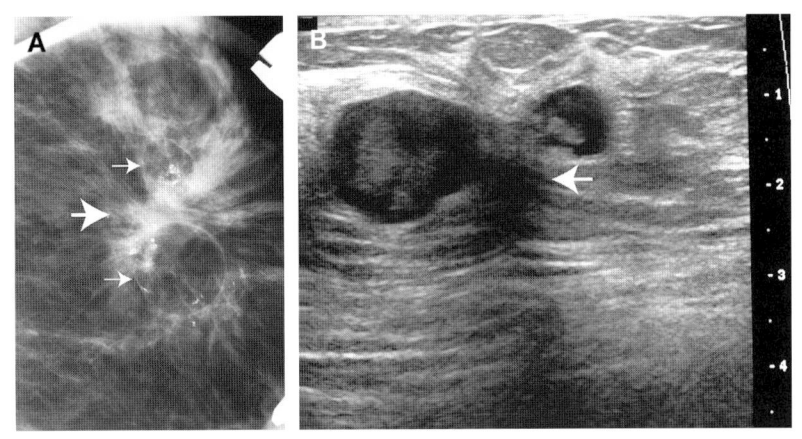

Fig. 8. Oil cysts and fat necrosis. (A) Spot-compression mammographic view of two oil cysts (*small arrows*) with associated dystrophic calcifications and an intervening spiculated mass (*large arrow*) caused by fat necrosis following reduction mammoplasty. (B) Ultrasound demonstrates two adjacent complex cystic masses, corresponding to the oil cysts seen mammographically, and an intervening area of distortion and shadowing (*arrow*), corresponding to the spiculated mass seen on mammography.

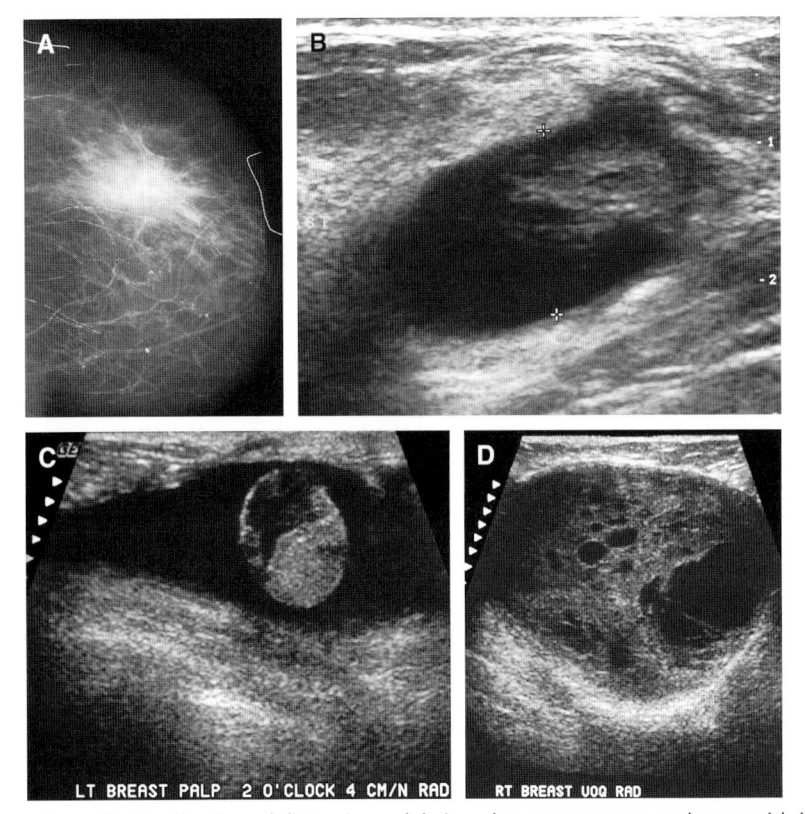

Fig. 9. Postlumpectomy fluid collections. (A) Craniocaudal view demonstrates an oval mass with indistinct margins corresponding to a known lumpectomy site. (B) Ultrasound demonstrates a complex cystic mass corresponding to the mammographic mass in (A). Such a cystic mass requires no further intervention unless the patient is symptomatic or a superimposed inflammatory process is suspected. In most patients, postoperative fluid collections resolve spontaneously. (C) Ultrasound in a patient who had a palpable postoperative fluid collection in the left breast in the 2:00 position, 4 cm from the nipple. The fluid collection was a complex cystic mass corresponding to a known lumpectomy site and was nearly anechoic with an associated mural nodule. Because the complex cystic mass corresponded directly with the lumpectomy site, a postoperative fluid collection could be diagnosed with confidence on the basis of sonography. On subsequent mammography and ultrasound, postoperative fluid collections may remain stable in appearance, decrease in size progressively, or even resolve completely. (D) Ultrasound demonstrates a complex cystic mass corresponding to a known lumpectomy site in the upper outer quadrant of the right breast. In this patient, the fluid collection has a more solid appearance with associated cystic spaces. This fluid collection requires no further intervention unless the patient is symptomatic or a superimposed inflammatory process is suspected.

submitting the aspirated fluid for cytologic examination, they perform core biopsies of the abnormality.

Cyst fluid contains a variety of electrolytes, proteins, and hormones [3]. On the basis of the electrolyte content and the cell lining, cysts can be separated into two primary groups: epithelial cell–lined cysts and cysts lined with cells characterized by apocrine metaplasia. Epithelial cell–lined cysts are characterized by fluid high in sodium and low in potassium, much like the composition of serum. It has been suggested that these cysts rarely recur after aspiration. Cysts lined with cells demonstrating apocrine metaplasia are characterized by fluid low in sodium and high in potassium. This electrolyte content suggests a more active cellular process leading to the concentration of potassium. It may be that these cysts recur after aspiration more commonly than do epithelial cell-lined cysts [3–5].

Oil cysts

On mammography, oil cysts appear as radiolucent or mixed-density masses (Fig. 8A). Oil cysts can be single or multiple, unilateral or bilateral. Oil cysts are variable in size and in some patients can resolve completely, as demonstrated on subsequent mammograms. Oil cysts are idiopathic or develop in areas of prior trauma or surgery (oil cysts are particularly common after reduction mammoplasty), probably representing end-stage fat necrosis. Some oil cysts develop mural calcifications in the form of egg shell calcifications (calcifications with a radiolucent center) or en phase calcifications, which have a coarse, irregular, curvilinear appearance. In most women, oil cysts are asymptomatic and are noted incidentally on screening mammography. Some patients who have oil cysts present with a discrete, hard mass that is confirmed to be an oil cyst mammographically. In this situation, it is important to assure the patient and the referring physician that the palpable finding is an oil cyst and that no intervention or follow-up is required. Although the diagnosis is made mammographically, and sonography is not indicated, it is important to note that the sonographic appearance of oil cysts is variable. Oil cysts may be anechoic with posterior acoustic enhancement, they may contain internal

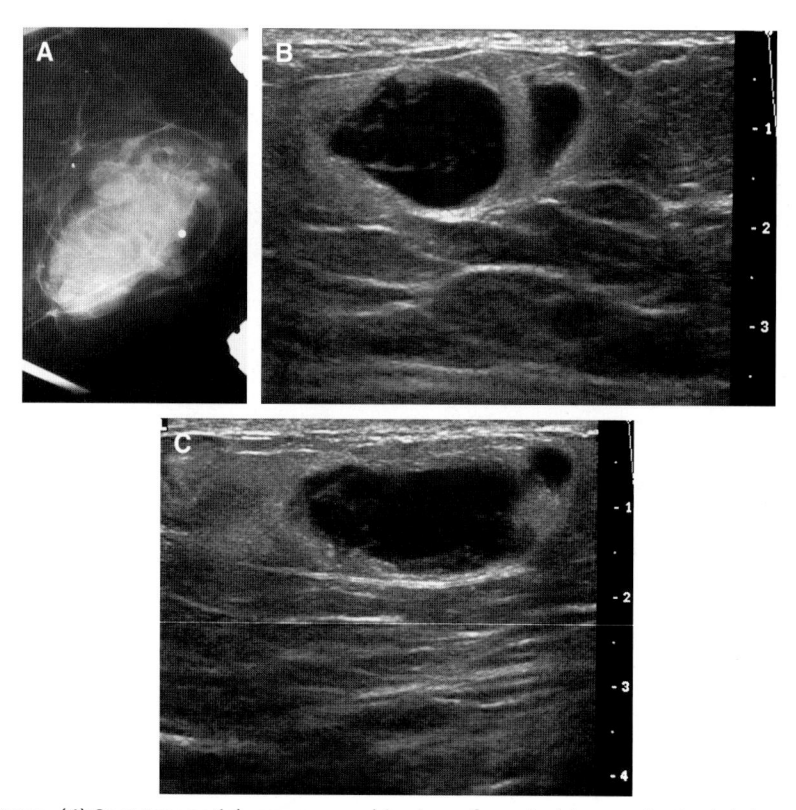

Fig. 10. Hematoma. (A) Spot tangential mammographic view of a palpable mass in the left breast in a patient describing the development of a "lump" after an automobile accident. A mixed-density mass is seen. (B and C) Ultrasound images through different portions of the mass demonstrate an area of hyperechoic tissue that is not well circumscribed and is associated with cystic spaces of variable size, characteristic of an evolving hematoma.

echoes, or they may contain intracystic solid-appearing components (Fig. 8B). Sometimes oil cysts appear solid and demonstrate shadowing.

In some women, oil cysts may demonstrate thickened, ill-defined, or spiculated margins or the presence of a round or oval soft tissue mass within a larger radiolucent (fatty) component on mammography. In such patients, if there is a history of breast trauma or surgery and if fat (radiolucency) is associated with the mass in two orthogonal mammographic projections, no intervention or short-term follow-up is warranted, even in the presence of spiculated margins or an associated nodule.

Other fluid collections

Other fluid collections seen in the breast include postoperative or traumatic fluid collections (eg, hematomas), galactoceles, and abscesses. The mammographic appearance of these lesions is variable. Round and oval masses with indistinct or ill-defined margins are common. Sonographically, these other fluid collections can appear as cystic, complex cystic, or, rarely, as solid masses.

Postoperative and traumatic fluid collections

Fluid collections in the breast may develop after surgery, particularly after lumpectomy and radiation therapy or trauma. In some patients, fluid collections resulting from surgery or trauma may appear indistinguishable from a simple cyst. In other patients, these fluid collections have a variable ultrasound appearance, which may include mural

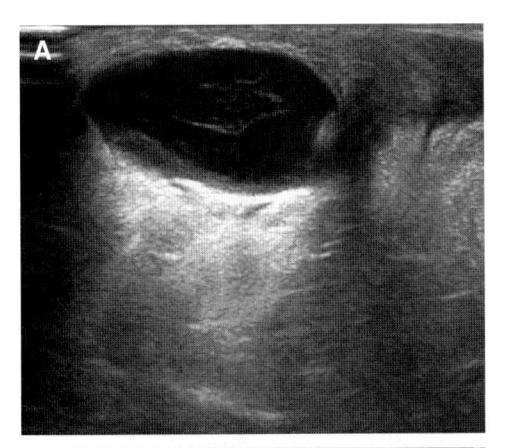

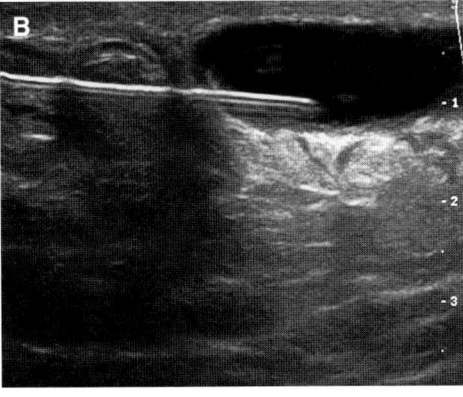

Fig. 11. Lactational abscess. (*A*) Ultrasound of a palpable, tender mass in the left breast in a patient who is lactating demonstrates a complex cystic mass with associated skin thickening. (*B*) An ultrasound-guided aspiration yielded 8 mL of purulent fluid. No residual abnormality was seen after aspiration. The patient was treated with oral antibiotics and experienced complete resolution of symptoms and no recurrence after completing antibiotic treatment.

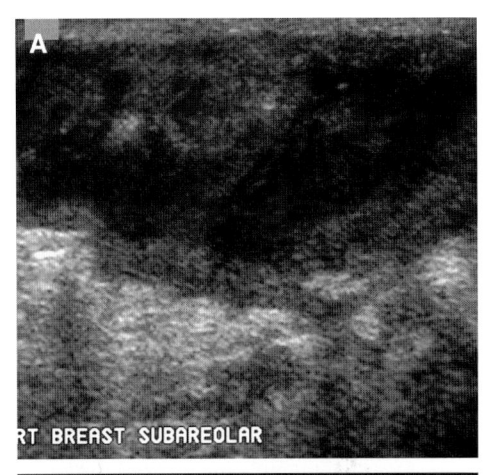

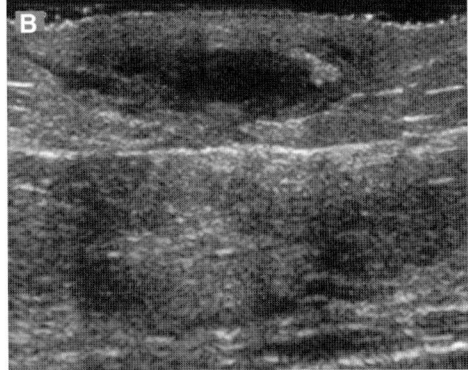

Fig. 12. Subareolar abscess. (*A*) Ultrasound in a patient presenting with a tender mass in the subareolar area demonstrates a complex cystic mass corresponding to the palpable finding. A small amount of purulent fluid was aspirated, and surgical drainage was performed. (*B*) Ultrasound in a different patient demonstrating a lenticular-shaped, hypoechoic mass associated with the dermal layer, consistent with a developing subareolar abscess. This appearance is common is the early stage of subareolar abscess development.

nodules, intracystic septations, or a combination of these features (Fig. 9). The walls may be irregular, lobulated, or thickened. It is important to recognize the benign nature of these fluid collections; unless infection is suspected, these collections should be left alone. Aspiration often leads to reaccumulation of fluid, and, rarely, aspiration may lead to the development of draining sinuses that can be difficult to treat.

On mammography, hematomas resulting from trauma may initially appear as soft tissue density masses; as hematomas liquefy and resolve, mixed-density masses may be seen (Fig. 10A). On ultrasound, hematomas resulting from trauma can appear as cystic or complex cystic masses; in some patients, an echogenic mass may be seen with associated cystic changes (Fig. 10B, C).

Galactoceles

Galactoceles are cysts that contain milky fluid and develop in women who are pregnant, lactating, or have stopped lactating within the last 2 to 3 years. On mammography, galactoceles appear as mixed-density or water-density masses. They often are indistinguishable from simple cysts, but they also can be associated with atypical features, including significant shadowing. On sonography, galactoceles appear as complex cystic masses, as solid-appearing masses, or as cysts. Fluid–fluid levels may be seen on mammography or sonography.

Abscesses

Patients who have breast abscesses can be divided into three groups: patients who have infections related to breastfeeding, patients who have recurring subareolar abscesses unrelated to nipple piercing or nipple rings, and patients who have peripheral mastitis or abscesses unrelated to pregnancy or lactation.

The author and colleagues most commonly see mastitis and breast abscesses in women who are breastfeeding ("puerperal mastitis"). These patients are usually treated by their obstetricians and are not referred for imaging. Mastitis reportedly occurs in approximately 2.5% of women who breastfeed, and abscess formation affects fewer than 1 in 15 women who breastfeed. In this patient population,

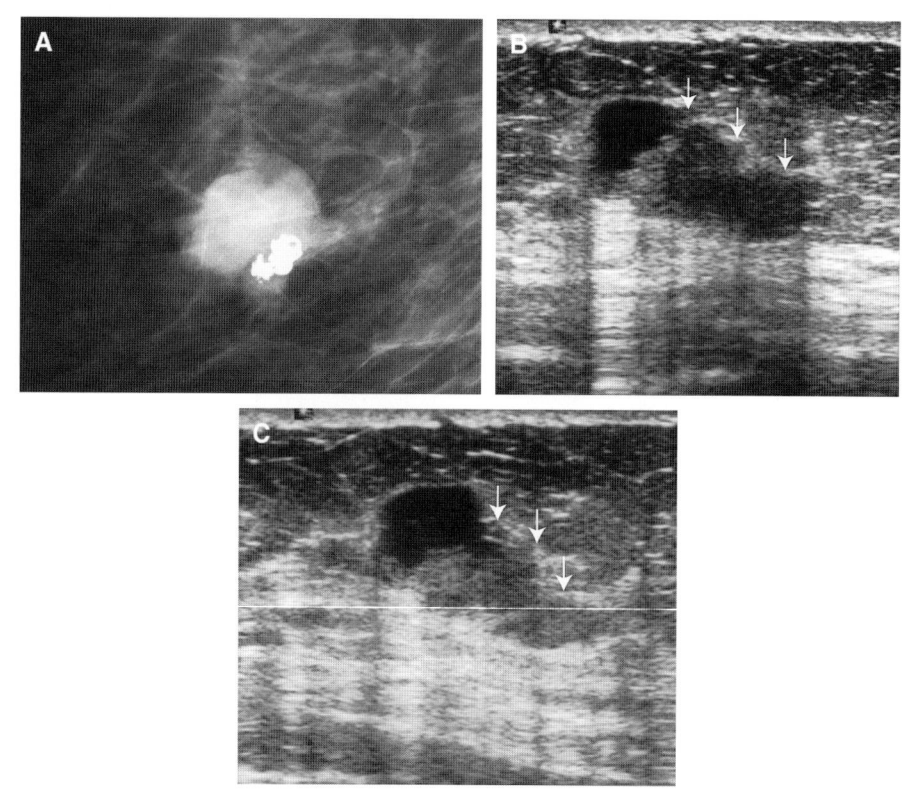

Fig. 13. Papilloma. (*A*) Craniocaudal mammographic view demonstrates a macrolobulated mass in the right breast with an associated coarse, dystrophic-type calcification. (*B* and *C*) Ultrasound images of the mass in the right breast demonstrate a soft tissue component (*arrows*) within a focally dilated duct. There is some associated posterior acoustic enhancement.

Staphylococcus aureus is the most common causative agent. Patients who have mastitis usually are treated effectively with antibiotics. If an abscess develops, percutaneous drainage can be helpful, and in some patients surgical drainage may be required. Patients do not need to stop breastfeeding during treatment and probably should be encouraged to continue. With abscess formation, a mass with ill-defined margins or spiculated margins and associated distortion may be seen on mammography. A complex cystic mass or, less commonly, an anechoic mass indistinguishable from a simple cyst may be seen on sonography (Fig. 11).

A second group of patients who have breast infections are those who have recurring subareolar abscess formation unrelated to nipple piercing or nipple rings. These patients are nonlactating, premenopausal women, usually with a history of heavy smoking. Some of these patients spontaneously develop periareolar fistulas (Zuska's disease). In such patients, squamous metaplasia involving the subareolar ducts is seen histologically. It is postulated that this process leads to obstruction of the ducts, with inspissation of secretions, duct wall erosion, and the development of periductal mastitis and abscess formation. Antibiotic therapy alone usually is not effective in these patients. Although some authors have advocated percutaneous drainage, this approach is not always effective. In most patients, wide surgical excision is required. In patients who undergo surgical drainage, there is a high incidence of recurrence. With recurrent episodes, the nipple begins to flatten, and some patients develop central horizontal inversion of the nipple. Bilateral abscess formation, either synchronous or metachronous, is seen in as many as 25% of patients who have recurrent subareolar abscess formation. It has been reported that these patients have a higher incidence of acne, hidradenitis suppurativa, and perineal inclusion cysts. Ultrasound in patients who have recurring subareolar abscesses demonstrates a complex cystic mass in the subareolar area (Fig. 12A). Early in the development of the abscess, ultrasound demonstrates a mass characterized by a lenticular shape, commonly associated with the dermal layer (Fig. 12B).

Peripheral mastitis or abscess formation also can be seen in women who are not pregnant or lactating. Rarely, patients who have such inflammations are diabetic; however, most of the women in this group are otherwise healthy with no identifiable source of infection. In this group of patients, a complex cystic mass usually is seen on sonography. These patients respond well to antibiotic therapy and usually do not experience a recurrence of the abscess. These women are also unlikely to present with bilateral abscesses.

Solitary papilloma

Solitary papillomas develop in subsegmental ducts. Women who have solitary papillomas commonly present with spontaneous nipple discharge. In these patients, ductography is helpful in establishing the presence, number, and the location of the lesions [6]. On mammography, papillomas can be identified as solitary masses or as clusters of round and punctate calcifications with or without an associated mass. Coarse, dense, curvilinear calcifications incidentally noted within dilated ductal structures or masses are also most likely sclerosed papillomas (Fig. 13A).

In patients who have solitary papillomas presenting with nipple discharge, ultrasound may reveal an intraductal lesion if the lesion is close to the nipple and there is associated ductal dilatation. Not all papillomas, however, are located close to the nipple or within dilated ducts. Therefore, normal ultrasound findings in a woman who has spontaneous

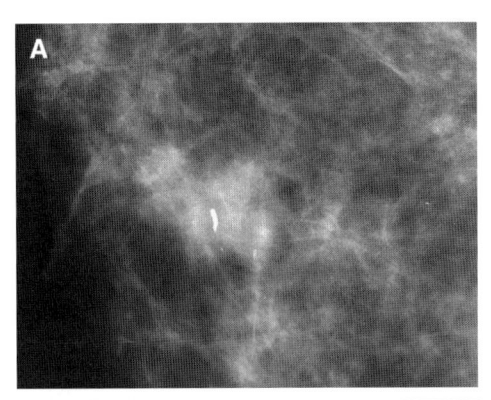

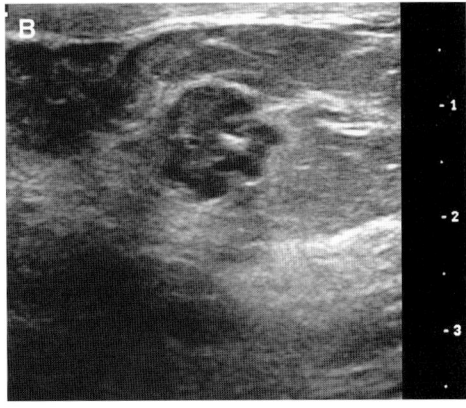

Fig. 14. Papilloma. (A) Craniocaudal mammographic view demonstrates an irregular mass with indistinct margins and an associated calcification. (B) Ultrasound demonstrates a complex cystic mass at the expected site of the mass seen mammographically. A linear high specular echo in the mass corresponds to the calcification seen on mammography.

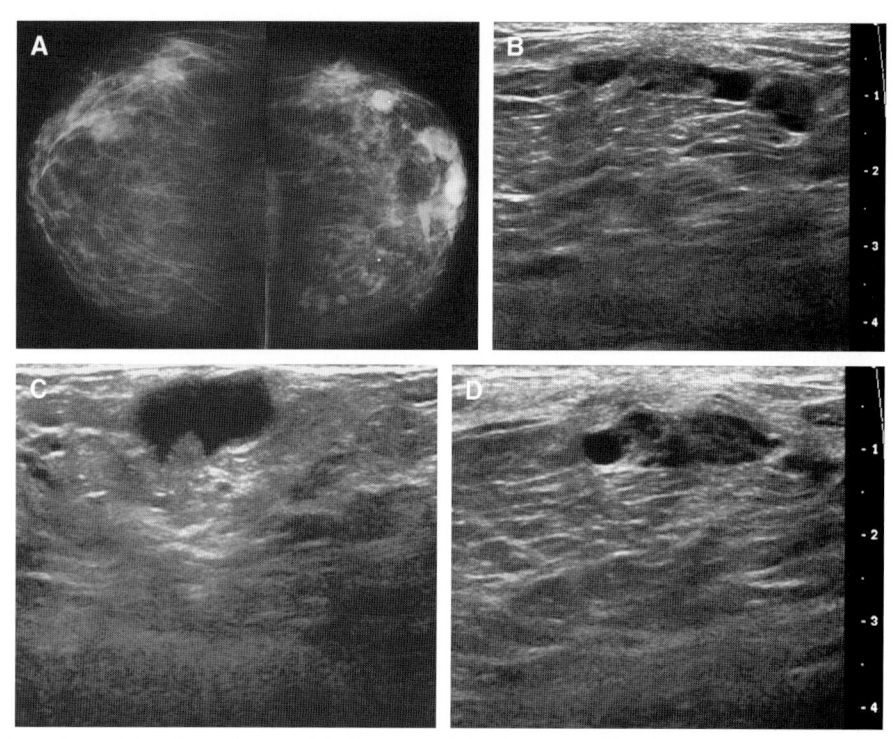

Fig. 15. Multiple peripheral papillomas. (*A*) Craniocaudal mammographic views demonstrate multiple masses of varying size and density in the left breast. (*B–D*) Ultrasound images demonstrate intraductal and intracystic lesions as well as complex cystic masses corresponding to some of the masses seen on mammography.

nipple discharge do not exclude the presence of a papilloma. Intraductal and intracystic papillomas are seen as soft tissue masses within dilated ductal structures (Fig. 13B, C) or as solid mural nodules within cysts. If a pneumocystogram is done after aspiration, the lesion can be outlined by air. A complex cystic mass (Fig. 14) or a homogeneously hypoechoic mass indistinguishable from other solid masses may be seen also.

Papillomas are small friable tumors with an epithelial lining contiguous with that of the duct. Therefore, papillomas are characterized by the presence of a contiguous layer of epithelial cells and a discontinuous basilar layer of myoepithelial cells. The presence of a central fibrovascular core distinguishes these lesions from epithelial hyperplasia with papillary changes, which is referred to as "papillomatosis" by some pathologists. Proliferative

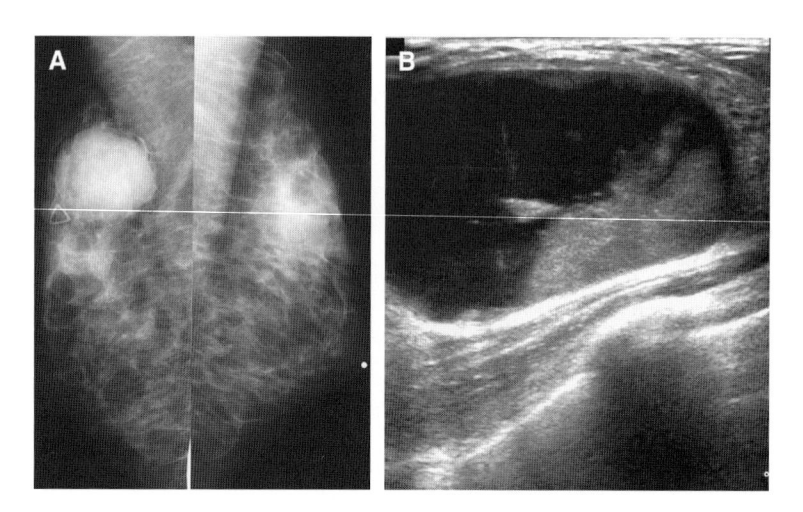

Fig. 16. Papillary carcinoma. (*A*) Mediolateral oblique mammographic views demonstrate a round mass in the right breast. The patient had no history of breast surgery or breast trauma. (*B*) Ultrasound demonstrates a complex cystic mass in the right breast corresponding to the mass seen mammographically.

changes, including hyperplasia, atypical hyperplasia, and ductal carcinoma in situ, may be seen in association with the epithelial lining of papillomas.

Multiple peripheral papillomas

Multiple peripheral papillomas develop in the terminal ducts. Histologically, these lesions are identical to solitary papillomas. Approximately 20% of women who have multiple peripheral papillomas present with spontaneous nipple discharge [7]. The other patients usually are asymptomatic and have papillomas detected on screening mammography. The mammographic findings in women who have multiple peripheral papillomas include lobulated masses, multiple peripheral masses of varying sizes, or unilateral or bilateral clusters of punctate calcifications [7]. On sonography, multiple solid masses or a combination of intracystic, intraductal, and solid masses may be seen (Fig. 15).

In contrast to patients who have solitary, central (ie, subareolar) papillomas, in whom the surrounding tissues often are unremarkable, patients who have multiple peripheral papillomas often have significant proliferative changes in the excised surrounding tissue, including atypical hyperplasia, lobular neoplasia, and ductal carcinoma in situ.

These changes are seen in up to 45% of patients, and, for this reason, some authors consider multiple peripheral papillomas to be markers of increased risk for development of breast cancer. The increased risk, if any, has not been quantified, however.

The management of multiple peripheral papillomas, particularly when they are regional or diffuse and bilateral, can pose a dilemma. The authors and colleagues' approach to patients who have localized multiple peripheral papillomas is excisional biopsy. In women who have more regional or diffuse findings, they recommend excision of any clinically symptomatic area or any lesion or lesions that change on follow-up mammography or ultrasound. After excisional biopsy of multiple peripheral papillomas, many patients present with recurrent lesions (new masses or calcifications at the site of the prior excision).

Some pathologists use the term "papillomatosis" to describe multiple peripheral papillomas (lesions with a central fibrovascular core), and others use the term to mean intraductal hyperplasia. The author thinks it is best to avoid the term "papillomatosis." When confronted with the term in a report, she asks the pathologist how the term is being used.

The care of patients diagnosed as having papillomas on core needle biopsy remains controversial

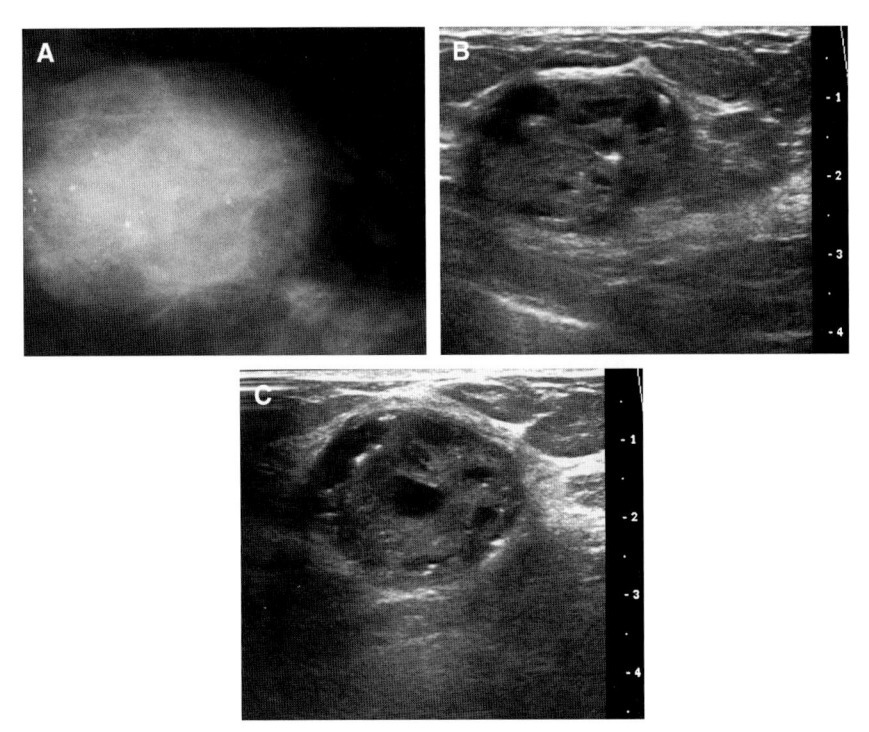

Fig. 17. Complex fibroadenoma. (*A*) Craniocaudal mammographic view demonstrates a dense mass with associated round and punctate calcifications. (*B* and *C*) Ultrasound images through different portions of the mass demonstrate a complex cystic mass with associated calcifications (high specular echoes).

[8–14]. Clearly, papillary lesions with atypia on core needle biopsy require excisional biopsy. In this group of patients, the rate of malignancy on excision is reported to be 31% to 60%. The controversy centers on what to do for patients who have a diagnosis of a benign papillary lesion with no associated atypia on core biopsy. Many authors advocate follow-up with no excision for patients without associated atypia, but other authors recommend excision of all papillary lesions regardless of the presence of associated atypia. In patients initially diagnosed with a papilloma and no associated atypia, the rate of malignancy on excision is reported to be 0% to 18% [8–14]. In evaluating the literature on papillary lesions, it is important to recognize that relatively few cases have been described, the studies are retrospective, and classification of lesions as central, usually solitary papillomas or multiple peripheral papillomas has been inadequate. In addition, the follow-up on many of these patients is limited; 2- to 3-year follow-up is probably insufficient to permit meaningful assessment of the biologic significance of many of these lesions.

As with so many other situations in breast imaging, the author and colleagues suggest that the clinical context is important in determining the appropriate management of papillary lesions. When a papilloma is diagnosed on core biopsy, the larger the lesion, the greater the number of abnormal findings, and the older the patient, the more appropriate an excisional biopsy seems. It may be that patients who have multiple peripheral papillomas should be treated more aggressively and that excisional biopsy is appropriate in such patients after an imaging-guided biopsy. In this context, it also is important to recognize that it may be difficult for the pathologist to distinguish

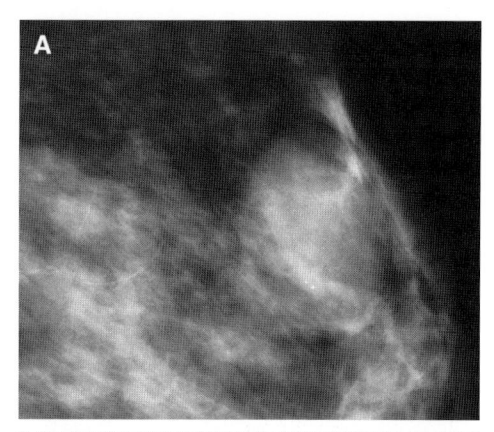

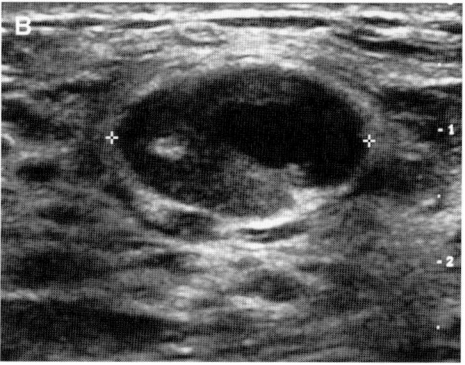

Fig. 18. Pseudoangiomatous stromal hyperplasia. (*A*) Spot-compression mammographic view confirms the presence of a round, well-circumscribed mass in the left breast. (*B*) Ultrasound demonstrates an oval, well-circumscribed complex cystic mass corresponding to the mammographic finding.

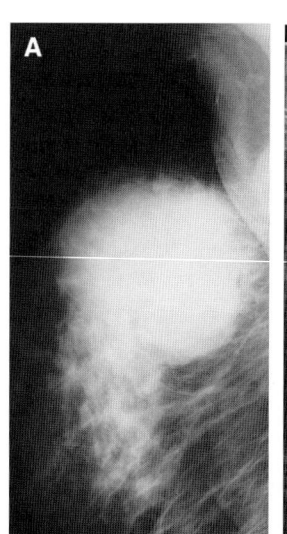

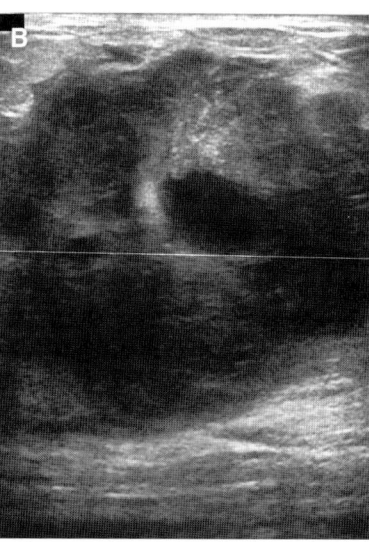

Fig. 19. Poorly differentiated invasive ductal carcinoma with necrosis. (*A*) Mediolateral oblique mammographic view demonstrates a round mass with indistinct margins in the right breast. Poorly differentiated infiltrating ductal carcinomas not otherwise specified commonly present as round masses on mammography. (*B*) Ultrasound demonstrates a round complex cystic mass with posterior acoustic enhancement, corresponding to the mammographic abnormality.

between benign papillomas, papillomas with atypia, and papillary carcinomas on review of core biopsy samples. As with the distinction between normal breast ductules and tubular carcinoma, the presence or absence of myoepithelial cells distinguishes benign from malignant papillary lesions. As much as 10% of a malignant papillary lesion has myoepithelial cells present, introducing the possibility of sampling bias.

Papillary carcinoma

Papillary carcinoma, which occurs as in situ and invasive variants, is common in older patients and accounts for 1% to 2% of all breast cancers [3–5]. As with papillomas, papillary carcinomas can occur in a central or a peripheral location. Patients who have central papillary carcinomas usually present with a palpable, well-circumscribed mass in the subareolar area. The mass may be large enough to cause nipple displacement and stretching of the overlying skin. Some of these patients may have associated nipple discharge. Bloody fluid often is obtained on aspiration. Patients who have peripheral papillary carcinomas (Fig. 16) can present with one or multiple masses with well-circumscribed to ill-defined but usually not spiculated margins. On ultrasound, a predominantly cystic but complex mass is the most common feature in papillary carcinoma [15,16]. Some papillary carcinomas are solid, however.

Complex cystic masses

Complex cystic masses can occur in a variety of circumstances. Although there can be significant overlap between categories, the author and colleagues characterize these masses as predominantly cystic with solid components or as predominantly solid with cystic components. Included in the predominantly cystic group are postoperative and traumatic fluid collections, oil cysts, abscesses, fat necrosis, galactoceles, papillomas, and papillary carcinomas.

In the predominantly solid group, the benign lesions include complex fibroadenomas (fibroadenomas with superimposed fibrocystic changes) (Fig. 17) [17], pseudoangiomatous stromal hyperplasia (Fig. 18); phyllodes tumors; galactoceles; chronic postoperative fluid collections; and fat necrosis in the acute setting, which often appears as a hyperechoic mass with cystic components. The malignant lesions in the predominantly solid group include invasive ductal carcinomas associated with necrosis (Fig. 19); papillary carcinomas; malignant phyllodes tumors; metastatic lesions; and, rarely, mucinous carcinomas.

References

[1] Mendelson EB, Tobin CE. Critical pathways in using breast US. Radiographics 1995;15(4): 935–45.
[2] Werner JK, Kumar D, Berg WA. Apocrine metaplasia: mammographic and sonographic appearance. AJR Am J Roentgenol 1998;170(5):1375–9.
[3] Elston CW, Ellis IO, editors. The breast. 3rd edition. Edinburgh (UK): Churchill Livingstone; 1998.
[4] Tavassoli FA. Pathology of the breast. 2nd edition. New York: McGraw Hill; 1999.
[5] Rosen PP. Rosen's breast pathology. 2nd edition. Philadelphia: Lippincott Williams and Wilkins; 2001.
[6] Cardenosa G, Doudna C, Eklund GW. Ductography of the breast: technique and findings. AJR Am J Roentgenol 1994;162(5):1081–7.
[7] Cardenosa G, Eklund GW. Benign papillary neoplasms of the breast: mammographic findings. Radiology 1991;181(3):751–5.
[8] Agoff SN, Lawton TJ. Papillary lesions of the breast with and without atypical ductal hyperplasia. Am J Clin Pathol 2004;122(3):440–3.
[9] Berg WA. Image-guided breast biopsy and management of high-risk lesions. Radiol Clin North Am 2004;42(5):935–46.
[10] Carder PJ, Garvican J, Haigh I, et al. Needle core biopsy can reliably distinguish between benign and malignant papillary lesions of the breast. Histopathology 2005;46(3):320–7.
[11] Ivan D, Selinko V, Sahin AA, et al. Accuracy of core needle biopsy diagnosis in assessing papillary breast lesions: histologic predictors of malignancy. Mod Pathol 2004;17(2):165–71.
[12] Jacobs TW, Connolly JL, Schnitt SJ. Nonmalignant lesions in breast core needle biopsies. Am J Surg Pathol 2002;26(9):1095–110.
[13] Mercado CL, Hamele-Bena D, Oken SM, et al. Papillary lesions of the breast at percutaneous core-needle biopsy. Radiology 2006;238(3): 801–8.
[14] Renshaw AA, Derhagopian RP, Tizol-Blanco DM, et al. Papillomas and atypical papillomas in breast core needle biopsy specimens. Am J Clin Pathol 2004;122(2):217–21.
[15] Schneider JA. Invasive papillary breast carcinoma: mammographic and sonographic appearance. Radiology 1989;171(2):377–9.
[16] Soo MS, Williford ME, Walsh R, et al. Papillary carcinoma of the breast: imaging finding. AJR Am J Roentgenol 1995;164(2):321–6.
[17] Dupont WD, Page DL, Parl FF, et al. Long-term risk of breast cancer in women with fibroadenoma. N Engl J Med 1994;331(1):10–5.

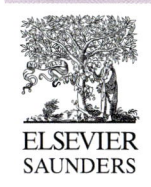

Sonography of Ductal Carcinoma in Situ

Beverly E. Hashimoto, MD

- Epidemiology of ductal carcinoma in situ
- Anatomy of ductal carcinoma in situ
- Ductal carcinoma in situ versus atypical ductal hyperplasia
- Ductal carcinoma in situ versus lobular carcinoma in situ and invasive cancer
- Important histopathologic prognostic features
- Bilaterality and multicentricity
- Mammographic appearance of ductal carcinoma in situ
- Sonographic technique for imaging ductal carcinoma in situ
- Sonographic appearances of ductal carcinoma in situ
  Calcifications
  Solid mass
  Solid mass associated with a fluid collection
  Abnormal duct
  Cluster of small cysts
- Sonographically guided interventional procedures
- Summary
- Acknowledgments
- References

Ductal carcinoma in situ (DCIS) was first recognized at the beginning of the twentieth century. Initially, DCIS was identified mainly along with invasive malignancy in mastectomy specimens, and the clinical significance of DCIS was not clear. Two long-term prospective studies, however, have followed patients who had untreated DCIS and have clarified the natural history of the disease [1,2]. These studies indicate that DCIS is a precursor to invasive carcinoma. DCIS evolves into invasive carcinoma over an average of 5 to 8 years. Between 25% and 50% of women who have untreated DCIS develop invasive carcinoma in the same breast quadrant. Among patients in whom DCIS is not completely removed surgically, 33% will have a recurrent neoplasm, and 50% of these recurrences will be invasive cancer. Page and colleagues has suggested that much of the survival advantage of screening mammography in younger women may result from the detection of DCIS [1,2]. Therefore, identification of DCIS continues to be an important goal for breast imagers.

Epidemiology of ductal carcinoma in situ

Before mammographic screening, DCIS was relatively uncommon. In 1973, the incidence of DCIS was 2.3 cases per 100,000 women. In the premammography era, DCIS was discovered as a palpable mass, Paget's disease, or nipple discharge. After the establishment of mammographic screening, the age-adjusted incidence of DCIS rose to 15.8 cases per 100,000 women in 1992, an increase of 587%. For comparison, the incidence of invasive cancer increased by 34.3% during the same period (1973–1992). The increase in the incidence of DCIS was demonstrated for white and African American women and for women younger than 50 years and women 50 years or older [3]. Furthermore, DCIS has become one of the most common

Virginia Mason Medical Center, 1100 Ninth Avenue, Seattle, WA 98101, USA
E-mail address: radbeh@vmmc.org

mammographically detected nonpalpable malignancies. A review of 21 studies published between 1989 and 1997 found that DCIS accounted for 39% of all malignant results from 13,125 biopsies of nonpalpable mammographic abnormalities [4]. Numerous autopsy studies have been performed to identify the natural prevalence of DCIS. These studies have shown prevalence rates between 0.2% and 18.2% [5]. Some of the differences are related to age, race, and possibly national origin [5]. Screening data indicate that the incidence of DCIS is higher in younger women than in older women. Researchers analyzing data from 653,833 mammograms performed by the National Cancer Institute's Breast Cancer Surveillance Consortium in 1996 and 1997 reported that DCIS accounted for 28.2% of screen-detected cancers in women aged 40 to 49 years and 16% of screen-detected cancers in women aged 70 to 84 years [3].

Given the increasing breast cancer screening of women under the age of 50 years and the greater incidence of DCIS in younger women, the detection rate of DCIS may continue to increase [4,6–8]. The average age of women at diagnosis of DCIS is about 10 years younger than the average age of women at diagnosis of invasive breast carcinoma. One study reported that 69% of all cases of DCIS were in premenopausal women [4].

Anatomy of ductal carcinoma in situ

To understand the imaging of DCIS, it is useful to understand the microscopic appearance of DCIS as well as the relationship between DCIS and its closely related pathologic entities.

The breast ductal system starts at the nipple. Between 15 and 25 lactiferous ducts extend from the nipple and branch into segmental, subsegmental, and terminal ducts. The terminal ducts are associated with lobules, with which they form terminal ductal-lobular units (TDLUs) [9]. In the normal breast, the terminal ducts and lobules are lined by one inner layer of epithelium and one outer layer of myoepithelium. Most breast malignancies arise within the TDLUs.

Ductal carcinoma in situ versus atypical ductal hyperplasia

When the epithelium of the TDLU proliferates, there is more than one layer of epithelial cells. This proliferation is called "epithelial hyperplasia." If multiple cell lines proliferate or clone themselves, the terminal duct or lobule becomes filled with a heterogeneous population of small cells. This result is called "typical" or "benign" epithelial hyperplasia. If the proliferating cells are uniform in appearance, the lesion is classified as either atypical ductal hyperplasia or grade 1 (low-grade) DCIS. The tumor is labeled atypical ductal hyperplasia if the abnormal proliferation is very small—that is, confined to only a part of the TDLU, involving no more than two TDLUs, and not larger than 2 mm [10]. If the tumor exceeds any of these parameters, it is labeled DCIS. Therefore, DCIS differs from atypical ductal hyperplasia only in terms of the size of the affected area.

Ductal carcinoma in situ versus lobular carcinoma in situ and invasive cancer

DCIS also may appear similar to lobular carcinoma in situ (LCIS) and some forms of invasive malignancy. LCIS, like DCIS, originates from the TDLUs, but the cells of LCIS are smaller, are less cohesive, and do not form papillary or glandlike patterns [11]. DCIS differs from invasive cancer in the appearance of the basement membrane. Whereas in invasive cancer the basement membrane is discontinuous or focally absent, in DCIS the basement membrane is intact.

Important histopathologic prognostic features

Microscopically, the important histopathologic prognostic features of DCIS are nuclear grade, presence or absence of central necrosis, cellular phenotypes, and growth pattern. Of these four parameters, nuclear grade is the most important. Low-grade cells usually are estrogen-receptor positive and have small monotonous nuclei with no or few mitoses. Intermediate-grade cells have mildly to moderately enlarged heterogeneous nuclei with few mitoses. High-grade cells usually are estrogen-receptor negative and have large, generally aneuploid nuclei with a high mitotic rate and irregular mitoses. Within a single DCIS lesion, there may be a variety of cellular grades; the accepted method is to classify the tumor according to the cells with highest nuclear grade [11].

The second most important histopathologic prognostic factor is the presence or absence of central necrosis in the ductal lumen. This necrotic material may calcify and form a cast of the duct and lobules. The presence of necrosis is important because the recurrence rate for DCIS with central necrosis is higher than the recurrence rate for DCIS without central necrosis. In one study in which DCIS lesions were smaller than 2.5 cm, the recurrence rate was 19% for DCIS with central necrosis, 10% for cribriform DCIS without necrosis, and 0% for micropapillary DCIS without necrosis [5].

Besides nuclear grade and central necrosis, the pathologist describes the cellular phenotypes of the tumor. Some examples of these phenotypes are apocrine DCIS, endocrine DCIS, clear cell DCIS, and signet-ring cell DCIS. These subtypes are important because they may affect the patient's treatment or posttreatment surveillance. Signet-ring cell DCIS associated with invasive malignancy has been shown to exhibit more aggressive behavior. Apocrine cell DCIS has a hormonal control mechanism that differs from the hormonal control mechanism of other more common malignancies. Whereas normal breast epithelial cells are immunoreactive for estrogen and progesterone receptors [12], apocrine cell DCIS is not immunoreactive for estrogen or progesterone receptors but does express androgen receptors [5]. Patients who have estrogen- and progesterone-receptor–negative tumors have been found to have shorter disease-free survival than patients who have estrogen- and progesterone-receptor–positive tumors [13]. Although tailored treatment options have not yet been developed, the presence of an apocrine cell population may affect the treatment plan.

Finally, the pattern of cellular growth is an important histopathologic feature that differentiates DCIS from other epithelial lesions such as atypical ductal hyperplasia and LCIS. The DCIS growth patterns include micropapillary, cribriform, solid, and clinging DCIS. The growth patterns are independent of nuclear grade and central necrosis: any of these growth patterns may exhibit high, intermediate, or low nuclear grade and may or may not be associated with central necrosis [11].

Bilaterality and multicentricity

Studies have reported a wide range of rates of DCIS coexisting with contralateral breast malignancies. The incidence rate ranges from 2.2% to 22% [5]. In these studies, the contralateral malignancy may be either DCIS or invasive malignancy. The wide range of rates may be result in part from differences in microscopic diagnostic criteria.

Most studies report a high rate of multicentricity for DCIS. The frequency ranges from 12% to 80%; the wide range results in part from differences in defining multicentricity. If multicentricity is defined as the presence of tumor foci in noncontiguous quadrants or at least 5 cm apart, the frequency is closer to 12%. If the terms "multicentricity" and "multifocality" are used interchangeably, the frequency is much higher. Most cases of DCIS are multifocal; that is, they have more than one lesion within a quadrant or a 5-cm radius. Careful pathologic examinations performed by Holland and colleagues [14] demonstrated that DCIS spreads contiguously to the same or adjacent ductal systems. The extension is not uniform, however, and there may be segments of the affected ducts that do not contain tumor [5,14]. This work and a later study performed by the Van Nuys group headed by Silverstein [15] confirmed that DCIS lesions should be excised with much wider margins than the 1-mm margin defined by the National Surgical Adjuvant Breast and Bowel Project, the group that operated the clinical trial establishing the efficacy of lumpectomy and radiation therapy for treatment of DCIS [16–18]. Silverstein and colleagues [15] found that if the surgical margin around a DCIS lesion was less than 10 mm, 45% of patients were found to have residual DCIS in the breast at re-excision [15,18].

Mammographic appearance of ductal carcinoma in situ

Mammographically, DCIS presents most commonly as calcifications alone. Studies have reported that 62% to 72% of DCIS lesions present as a cluster of calcifications, 12% to 30% present as calcifications with a mammographic density or a circumscribed mass, and 10% to 12% present as a mass without calcifications. Researchers have found that mammographic masses presenting at the same time as DCIS correspond microscopically to either tumor or associated fibrosis [6]. Rare mammographic presentations of DCIS include architectural distortion and dilated ducts (either subareolar or distal to the nipple) [6,19–23]. In 6% to 15% of cases, DCIS is detected not mammographically but as an incidental finding in a biopsy specimen or in breast tissue removed during a cosmetic procedure [20,24,25].

Although the finding of clustered calcifications on mammography is extremely sensitive for the diagnosis of DCIS, the specificity of this finding is only 10% to 35% [26–33]. As a result of this relatively low specificity, about 60% to 80% of breast biopsies in patients who have mammographic calcifications are associated with benign histologic results [2,34–38]. Furthermore, mammography commonly does not demonstrate the size of the DCIS lesion accurately. The calcifications may not define the entire histologic extent of the disease, particularly in the case of low-grade DCIS [39]. This information is important because many patients who have DCIS are treated with local excision, and complete removal of this lesion is a key factor in preventing recurrence [40]. Therefore, the diagnosis and staging of DCIS remains a common radiographic problem.

Sonographic technique for imaging ductal carcinoma in situ

High-resolution sonography is necessary to demonstrate breast microcalcifications. Generally, frequencies higher than 10 MHz should be used. In addition to higher frequency, other sonographic parameters may improve the resolution of the image. One should be careful to optimize the focal zones for the region of interest. Increasing the line density and the persistence also will improve the resolution but will reduce the frame rate. If one has already identified a specific small lesion, a slow frame rate may not compromise the examination. For thicker breasts, harmonic imaging may produce high-resolution images at greater depths.

In addition to resolution, one should optimize image contrast. Because DCIS lesions are small and commonly isoechoic with fat, high-contrast imaging may improve visualization of these subtle lesions. The easiest method to increase the contrast is to reduce the dynamic range. Most machines have a variety of gray-scale maps. The sonologist should check the effect of these maps when a subtle mass is identified and choose the one that best emphasizes the differences in gray scale between fat and lesions isoechoic to fat. High-edge enhancement improves characterization of margins and delineation of duct walls. Spatial or frequency compounding produces improved contrast enhancement, which may improve visualization of masses.

Color and power Doppler imaging are useful techniques, particularly in clarifying the vascularity of clustered microcysts, possible intraductal masses, and thickened duct walls. One commonly overlooked parameter that strongly affects color or power Doppler sensitivity is the Doppler frequency. In general, the Doppler frequency should be about 2 to 4 MHz lower than the scanning frequency. Thus, if one is scanning with a gray-scale center frequency of 14 MHz, a color or power Doppler frequency of about 12 to 10 MHz should be used. Once the frequency is adjusted, the overall color or power Doppler gain should be increased until the entire image is filled with color. Once the image is obscured by color, the gain should be reduced slowly until the color barely clears the screen. The overall gain should remain at this level throughout the examination. If color or power Doppler is still not identified in normal breast tissues, the Doppler scale should be reduced until flecks of color are seen. If color or power Doppler sensitivity still needs to be improved, the wall filter can be reduced. Reduction of the wall filter increases flash in the image. Flash usually is not a significant problem in the breast. The most common causes of flash are respiration and cardiac motion, which has the biggest impact on the left breast. By instructing the patient to hold her breath briefly, the sonologist can reduce virtually all of the flash in the right breast and much of the flash in the left breast.

Finally, to maximize the sensitivity of color and power Doppler, the size of the gate can be increased. The gate controls the color pixel size, so that with a large gate, the color pixels are larger, and the color or the power Doppler resolution is poorer. Poor color or power Doppler resolution is not acceptable in some clinical situations. For example, in sonography of the carotid arteries, color may bleed into the adjacent tissues. In the breast, however, the blood vessels are much smaller, and poor color or power Doppler resolution does not compromise the examination. Because these blood vessels in the breast are small, a large gate increases the sensitivity of the color or the Doppler examination by potentially increasing the color or the Doppler signal for every pixel.

Although DCIS masses generally are not associated with movement, cine clips sometimes are useful to document the relationships between multiple abnormalities. For example, clips may be useful to show the relationship between multiple abnormal masses or the relative positions of abnormal ducts and masses. Cine clips also may enhance color or power Doppler imaging. Cine clips of color or power Doppler may clarify the location of blood flow within a mass or a septation. With a single real-time image, it sometimes is difficult to differentiate artifactual color signal from real color or power Doppler signals resulting from blood flow.

Wide field-of-view, three-dimensional, and four-dimensional sonographic imaging are being used increasingly within the breast. These techniques are particularly useful to characterize large masses or to delineate long intraductal spread of DCIS. The main limitation of these techniques for DCIS is that DCIS lesions generally are very small, and these techniques do not have the resolution to demonstrate microcalcifications or intraductal abnormalities reliably. The resolution of these techniques is improving, however, and in the future they may be useful for staging and surgical planning [41,42].

Sonographic appearances of ductal carcinoma in situ

There are five general sonographic appearances of DCIS: (1) calcifications, (2) solid mass, (3) solid mass associated with a fluid collection, (4) cluster of cysts, and (5) dilated ducts.

Calcifications

On mammography, DCIS most often presents as calcifications. Studies have shown that about two thirds of all mammographically identified DCIS lesions present as calcifications suggestive of malignancy [5,6]. Historically, sonography was not considered a useful diagnostic modality for DCIS because early studies showed that sonography had a poor sensitivity in the identification of calcifications [43–45]. With the low-frequency transducers that were previously used, researchers estimated that sonography was able to identify benign calcifications larger than 3 mm but could not reliably resolve calcifications smaller than 2 mm [46]. Malignant microcalcifications are often smaller than 0.5 mm [47].

Improvements in sonographic technique, including the introduction of higher-frequency transducers and more gray-scale contrast techniques, have allowed breast imagers to identify breast structural anatomy in much greater detail than was possible in the past. Researchers have shown, in vitro and in vivo, that by using a high-frequency transducer (at least 10 MHz), it is possible to identify calcifications 1 mm or smaller [48]. Even with high frequencies, improved software resolution, and improved contrast techniques, however, sonography still does not identify calcifications as well as mammography does. When mammography is used as the imaging standard, most researchers within the last 8 years have reported that the accuracy of sonography in the identification of breast calcifications is between 60% and 100%. The higher values tend to be associated with smaller studies. Even when calcifications are visible, sonography does not have the resolution to characterize the individual calcification shapes. The calcifications may be surrounded by normal-appearing breast tissue, may be within a solid mass, or may be within a duct (Fig. 1) [48–51].

Although the rate of detection of calcifications is lower for sonography than for mammography, sonographic evaluation of mammographic calcifications may be useful. Sonographic evaluation may provide additional information about the nature of the mammographic calcifications. Sonographic identification of mammographic calcifications is associated with a higher probability of malignancy. Sonographically, imagers uniformly identify malignant calcifications more commonly than benign calcifications. In one study, researchers found calcifications on sonography in 100% of malignant invasive masses, in 100% of DCIS lesions, and in 66% of benign lesions [50]. Another study, which correlated the sonographic findings with findings on microscopic examination of the tissue

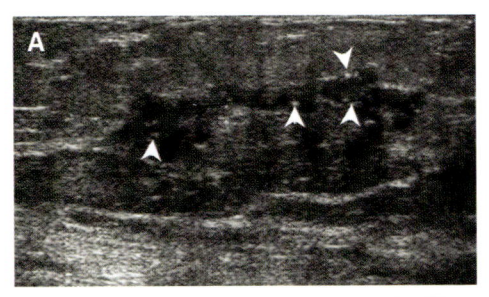

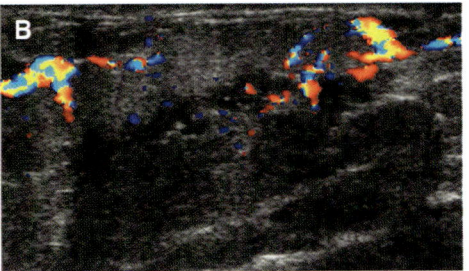

Fig. 1. An 88-year-old woman presented with bloody discharge from the left breast. A mammogram of the left breast demonstrated a cluster of calcifications at 9:00. (*A*) Radial sonography of the left breast at 9:00 demonstrated multiple clusters of calcifications (*arrowheads*), which appeared to be within irregular ducts. (*B*) Radial color Doppler sonography of the left breast at 9:00 showed increased vascularity in the area of the abnormal calcifications. The final diagnosis was high-grade DCIS with necrosis. Increased vascularity on color Doppler is commonly identified with high-grade DCIS.

specimens, found that the sonographic identification of calcifications in patients who have DCIS is more common in DCIS with necrosis than in DCIS without necrosis [52]. Therefore, sonographic identification of calcifications strengthens the probability that the mammographic calcifications represent a malignancy.

Solid mass

Although sonography may not identify mammographic calcifications themselves, imagers commonly identify masses on sonography in the region where calcifications were identified on mammography. Many researchers have found that in this circumstance, a sonographic mass corresponds to a higher probability of malignancy, either DCIS or invasive tumor [50,51].

A solid mass is the most common sonographic manifestation of DCIS (Fig. 2). Studies report the presence of a solid mass on sonography in 90% to 100% of DCIS cases. These high rates result from the selection of patients in these series. Many of these studies are biased toward larger tumors because the DCIS cases are from symptomatic patients or are identified retrospectively on the basis of results of ultrasound-guided biopsy. Even with this bias, however, the results from these studies are remarkably consistent. When a sonographic mass is evident, the calcifications seen on mammography may or may not be associated with a mass or asymmetry on mammography. Sonographically, solid masses in patients who have DCIS are either isoechoic or hypoechoic to fat, and they are round, oval, or irregular in shape. Investigators correlating the histologic findings with the sonographic appearance in patients who have DCIS have found that intermediate-grade DCIS tends to be round or oval, whereas high-grade DCIS tends to be irregular in shape [51,52]. The sonographic appearance is not a sure predictor of cellular grade, however, and grade must be confirmed by microscopic examination of the tumor [49,52,53].

The margins of DCIS masses can appear circumscribed or not circumscribed. If a mass is not circumscribed, the margins may be indistinct, angular, microlobulated, or spiculated. If a mass is well defined, it will not have a thin hyperechoic capsule, and it will be associated with heavy shadowing, no posterior acoustic effect, or a combined pattern—most commonly edge shadowing. Masses sometimes affect the surrounding tissues by distorting Cooper's ligaments or compressing tissue planes. Calcifications may or may not be present. Masses commonly exhibit intraductal extension [53–58]. Architectural distortion is associated mainly with high-grade DCIS, which may incite a surrounding inflammatory response [5].

When DCIS appears as a well-defined round or oval mass, it may be erroneously classified as American College of Radiology Breast Imaging and Reporting Data System (BI-RADS) category 3, probably benign. To avoid this error, a transducer frequency of at least 10 MHz should be used. The higher frequency allows identification of subtly indistinct margins. In general, however, even when the sonographic appearance of DCIS is equivocal, the mammographic appearance usually is suggestive of malignancy: the lesion has suspicious calcifications, or there is a mass or asymmetry with ill-defined or partially obscured margins on mammography.

A variant of the hypoechoic solid mass is an ill-defined region of generalized decreased acoustic

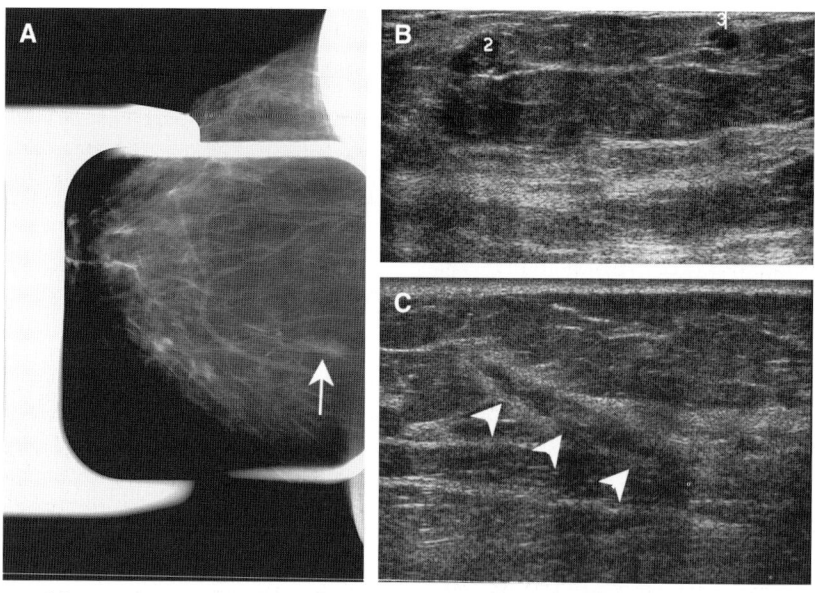

Fig. 2. A 73-year-old woman presented with a new asymmetry on screening mammography. (*A*) A right craniocaudal mammogram showed a focal asymmetry in the posterior medial breast (*arrow*). This mass could not be identified sonographically, so it was biopsied using mammographic stereotactic technique. (*B*) Radial sonography of the right breast at 2:00 demonstrated two solid masses (*2* and *3*) that were mammographically occult. These masses were biopsied with sonographic guidance. (*C*) Because all three masses were within the same quadrant, lumpectomy was planned. The surgeon requested that each mass be localized with intraoperative sonographic guidance alone (ie, localization without wire localization). Because the stereotactic biopsy tract (*arrowheads*) and the biopsy site were easily identified, all three lesions were localized with intraoperative sonographic guidance without the use of wires. The final diagnosis was low-to-intermediate grade DCIS without necrosis.

transmission. This appearance was described with early gray-scale technique but also has been documented with modern equipment (Fig. 3). This phenomenon is associated with a relatively large area of tissue, such as half a quadrant. The glandular tissue architecture appears either normal or uniformly filled with mildly dilated ducts. The abnormal region exhibits less acoustic transmission than seen in adjacent normal tissues, similar to that seen with benign inflammatory or edematous conditions. In the reported cases of ill-defined regions of decreased acoustic transmission [49,54,57,59], the imaging findings were subtle. The disease was discovered after the patient presented with an associated nipple discharge, lump, or firmness. Mammographically, these regions corresponded to ill-defined asymmetries. Calcifications were present in some cases but not in others. Ductography may demonstrate numerous small intraductal filling defects. MR imaging showed regional enhancement in some cases and segmental enhancement in others [49,54,57,59].

Solid mass associated with a fluid collection

The third sonographic appearance of DCIS is a solid mass associated with a fluid collection. The fluid collection usually is round or oval but may be irregular in shape. Solid masses within dilated ducts are included in this category. The most common type of tumor with this sonographic presentation is a benign lesion, but DCIS involving papillary lesions and a variety of histologic subtypes of DCIS also may present in this manner.

In the literature, papillary lesions and the papillary form of DCIS often are confused with one another. The papillary or micropapillary subtype of DCIS appears microscopically as small tufts of epithelium projecting into the wall of the duct lumen.

If there is asymmetric involvement of the luminal wall, this form of DCIS may appear as an intraductal mass on sonography. Papillary lesions, like DCIS, are epithelial masses that project into the ductal lumen. Unlike DCIS, papillary lesions contain a fibrovascular stalk.

Papillary tumors commonly represent benign papillomas, but these lesions may give rise to DCIS. Papillary lesions that give rise to DCIS exhibit the same variety of subtypes as normal epithelium [5,12]. Some authors refer to all DCIS in papillary lesions as "papillary DCIS" rather than describing the true subtype. Because papillary lesions commonly appear as intracystic or intraductal masses, DCIS associated with these masses generally is sonographically indistinguishable from benign papillomas.

Numerous studies have examined the frequency of associated malignancy in papillomas. In general, the frequency has been found to be 0.4% to 8%. Because papillomas seem to be associated with epithelial proliferation, most surgeons excise these lesions to exclude the presence of adjacent DCIS or invasive malignancy [5].

Abnormal duct

The fourth sonographic appearance of DCIS is an abnormal duct. The imager may identify only one or many abnormal ducts. The duct may be uniformly dilated or focally dilated (Fig. 4). A duct sometimes contains ill-defined amorphous material (similar to gallbladder sludge) or calcifications. In unusual cases, there is asymmetric thickening of the duct walls. If there are numerous abnormal ducts, they are within a segment or a region of the breast [54,56].

The sonographic appearance of abnormal ducts reflects the anatomic features of DCIS. Because

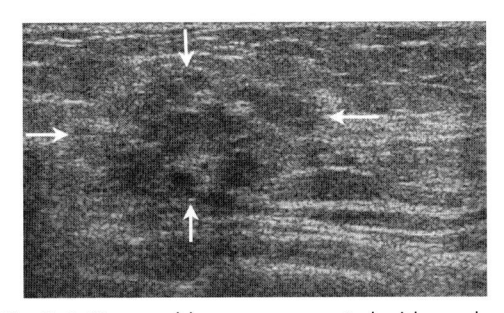

Fig. 3. A 42-year-old woman presented with a palpable abnormality in the left breast. On sonography of the left breast, there was an ill-defined area of hypoechogenicity (*arrows*) in the area of the palpable abnormality. The edges of this area blended into the adjacent fibroglandular tissue. This mass had intermittent shadowing. The final diagnosis was low-grade DCIS.

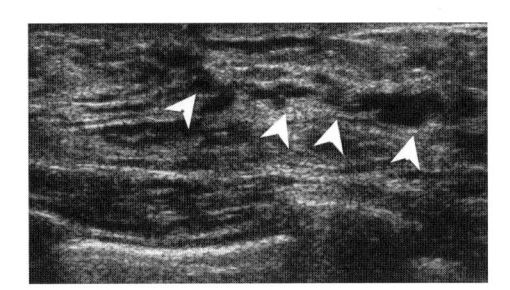

Fig. 4. A 46-year-old woman had abnormal calcifications on screening mammography of the right breast. On radial sonography of the right breast, there were abnormal, irregularly dilated ducts (*arrowheads*) in the area of the calcifications noted on mammography. No calcifications were identified on ultrasound. The final diagnosis was high-grade DCIS with necrosis.

DCIS starts in the TDLUs of the breast, the tumor commonly quickly fills the contiguous ducts. The tumor also may leave the TDLU and extend into adjacent ducts. Aggressive high-grade DCIS may form new ducts and fill them with malignant cells. The tumor dilates the ducts and produces calcifications, masses, and necrosis [11].

A clinical variant of abnormal ducts is ductal dilatation associated with an invasive malignancy (Figs. 5, 6). If a breast imager identifies a dilated duct or multiple dilated ducts extending from a sonographic mass suggestive of malignancy, the imager should suspect that the dilated ducts represents DCIS extending from the tumor. Usually, the dilated ducts are located on the side of the mass nearest the nipple, so they are best identified in the radial plane. If the mass is several centimeters from the nipple, the dilated ducts should be followed to see if any other irregular masses are associated with these abnormal tubular structures. If other masses are identified, these should be considered suggestive of other sites of invasive malignancy [60].

Cluster of small cysts

The final sonographic appearance of DCIS is a cluster of small cysts ("clustered microcysts") (Fig. 7).

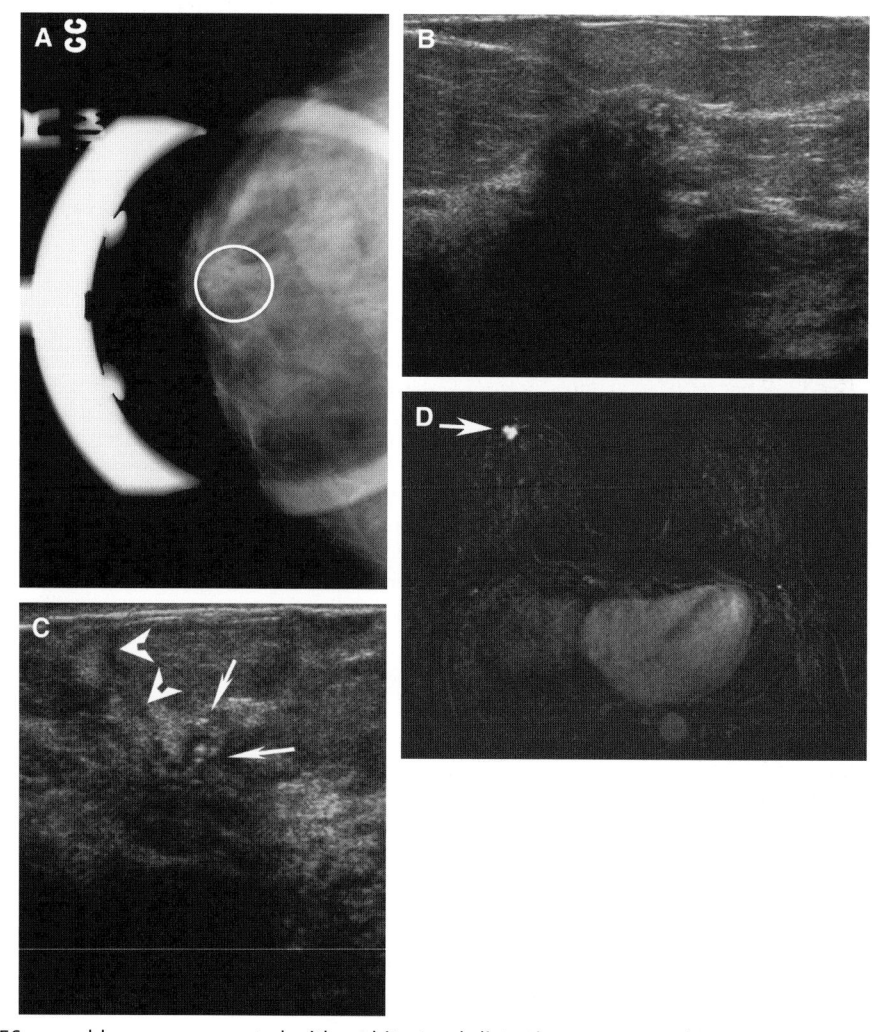

Fig. 5. A 56-year-old woman presented with architectural distortion on a screening mammogram of her right breast. (A) On a craniocaudal spot-compression view of the right breast, there was spiculated architectural distortion in the subareolar area (*circle*). (B) On sonography of the right breast, an irregular, hypoechoic, heavily shadowing mass was visible in the area of the spiculated lesion noted on mammography. (C) Adjacent to the sonographic mass in (B) were some dilated ducts (*arrowheads*) filled with calcifications (*arrows*). (D) MR imaging demonstrated an early enhancing right breast mass (*arrow*) that corresponded to the mass identified on mammography and ultrasound. The final diagnosis of the mass was invasive malignancy with ductal and lobular features. The dilated ducts and calcifications corresponded to adjacent high-grade DCIS with necrosis.

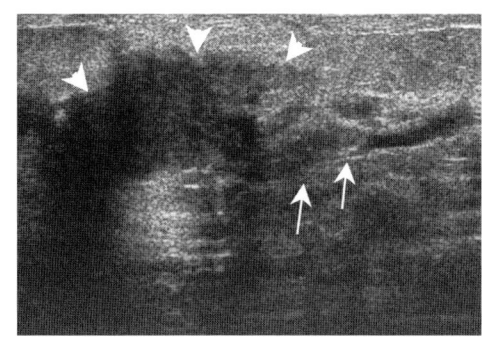

Fig. 6. A 65-year-old woman presented with a palpable abnormality in the right breast. Radial sonography of the right breast demonstrated that the palpable abnormality corresponded to an irregular, hypoechoic, solid mass (*arrowheads*). Extending from the mass was a tongue of tissue that filled a dilated duct (*arrows*). This ductal extension was characteristic of DCIS extending from the main tumor. The diagnosis on the basis of ultrasound-guided core needle biopsy of the mass was high-grade DCIS.

This finding is extremely uncommon. Most centers still classify clustered microcysts as BI-RADS category 3, probably benign, and recommend short-term sonographic follow-up, generally 6 months after the initial discovery.

There are a few clues that differentiate DCIS from benign clustered microcysts. DCIS in clustered microcysts tends to be more vascular than benign clustered microcysts. Therefore, one should apply the most sensitive color Doppler techniques to any clustered microcystic mass. If there is vascularity within or around the mass, biopsy probably is warranted. Microcysts associated with DCIS tend to have thicker, more irregular walls than benign microcysts. Commonly, the walls of benign clustered microcysts are so thin that they cannot be resolved. Even when the walls are visible, they do not produce highly specular reflections. Instead, there are tiny anechoic oval or round fluid structures connected together in the overall shape of a round or an oval mass. Microcysts associated with DCIS tend to be more irregular in shape and size than benign clustered microcysts. Whereas benign

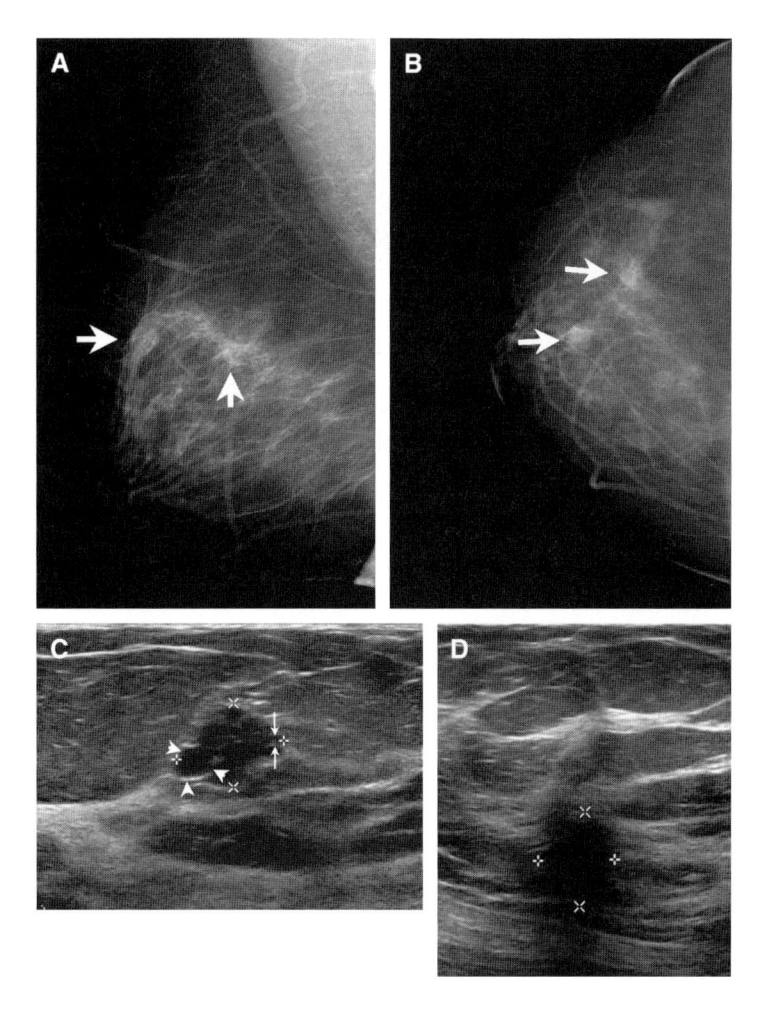

Fig. 7. A 59-year-old woman presented for screening mammography. (*A*) A mediolateral oblique mammogram and (*B*) a craniocaudal mammogram of the right breast demonstrated two abnormalities: a lobular mass at 12:00 and a cluster of calcifications at 10:00 (*arrows*). (*C*) Sonography of the right breast at 10:00 showed a cluster of cysts corresponding to the lobular mass identified on mammography. Unlike benign clusters of cysts, these cysts were unequal in size. For example, the arrowheads outline a large cyst, and the arrows denote a small cyst. (*D*) Sonography of the right breast at 12:00 demonstrated a solid, irregular, shadowing mass, corresponding to the location of the calcifications seen on mammography. The final diagnoses were DCIS at 10:00 and infiltrating ductal and lobular carcinoma at 12:00.

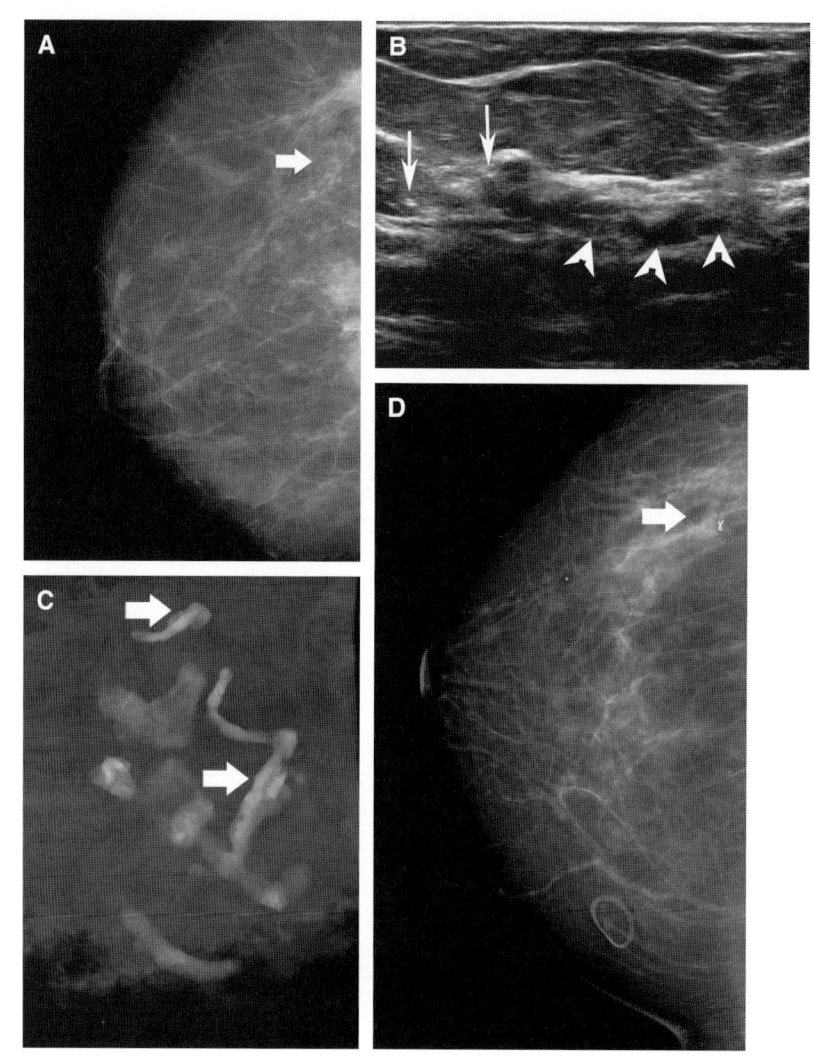

Fig. 8. A 66-year-old woman had calcifications suggestive of malignancy on mammography. (*A*) A craniocaudal mammogram of the right breast demonstrated a cluster of heterogeneous calcifications in the outer periphery of the breast (*arrow*). (*B*) Sonography of the right breast revealed irregularly dilated ducts (*arrowheads*) with calcifications (*arrows*) in the area of the calcifications noted on mammography. (*C*) A specimen radiograph obtained by vacuum-assisted ultrasound-guided 12-gauge biopsy performed on the dilated ducts demonstrated multiple calcifications (*arrows*). (*D*) A craniocaudal mammogram of the right breast demonstrated the sonographically placed clip (*arrow*). The presence of calcifications on specimen radiography and the clip placement confirmed that the site of the ultrasound-guided biopsy correlated well with the site of the calcifications identified on mammography. The final diagnosis was high-grade DCIS with necrosis.

microcysts are uniform in size and round or oval, microcysts associated with DCIS may be slightly flattened or non-uniform in size. These findings are extremely subtle, however, so careful short-term follow-up is important for any clustered microcysts [61,62].

Sonographically guided interventional procedures

Although DCIS features such as calcifications generally are best localized and biopsied mammographically, mammographic guidance may be difficult in certain clinical situations. For example, lesions in the extreme breast periphery or in the axilla may not be biopsied readily with standard mammographic or stereotactic techniques. In unusual situations, patients who have severe arthritis, recent abdominal or chest surgery, or severe vasovagal reactions may not be able to undergo procedures that require that the patient be in a prone or a sitting position. In these circumstances, sonographic guidance is extremely useful as long as the lesion can be identified sonographically.

If a lesion suggestive of DCIS can be visualized sonographically, many of the sonographic interventional procedures used for other breast abnormalities can be performed. The most common procedures are sonographically guided core needle biopsy and sonographically guided needle localization [63]. When DCIS presents as a mass, with or without an associated fluid collection, it usually is possible to perform a standard 14-gauge core needle biopsy. If calcifications are present, and there is a need to correlate the sonographic findings with mammographic calcifications, a clip may be placed after the biopsy is performed. A postbiopsy specimen radiograph determines whether the calcifications are within the resection specimen, and postprocedural mammograms confirm that the clip is in the same location as the mammographic calcifications. If no calcifications are present within the specimen, more cores may be obtained to ensure that adequate material has been obtained. The additional cores should also be radiographed to confirm the presence of calcifications (Fig. 8).

For DCIS that presents as abnormal ducts, isolated calcifications, or extremely small masses (< 5 mm), one may consider a larger-gauge core biopsy. Vacuum-assisted core biopsy systems produce much larger (11- and 12-gauge) cores. The main disadvantage is that these larger needle systems sometimes are more difficult to maneuver into position for biopsy [54].

Needle localization is another common interventional technique performed with sonographic guidance. If a lesion is easily visible, and the surgeon is experienced or has confidence in the sonologist, the lesion can be localized intraoperatively without a wire. With this technique, one identifies the location of the DCIS tumor after the patient has been anesthetized. The location of the tumor can be marked on the skin before cleansing of the skin, or the sonographic transducer can be covered with a sterile cover, and the tumor can be identified on the sterile field. When the surgeon is aware of the relative position and the size of the tumor under the skin, the surgeon can excise down to the lesion and perform the lumpectomy (see Fig. 2) [64].

If sonographic needle localization is preferred, one can use the same needle guidewire systems that are used for standard mammographically guided needle localizations. This procedure may be performed for DCIS masses and also for subtle lesions that have been biopsied initially using stereotactic technique. As long as the previous stereotactic biopsy was performed within a few weeks of the surgery date, sonographic needle localization usually can be performed, because the biopsy cavity is generally easily visible. After sonographically guided needle localization, one should obtain craniocaudal and 90° lateral mammograms to confirm that the needle location correlates with the mammographic abnormality [58,63].

Summary

With the improved sonographic imaging techniques are now available, radiologists can use ultrasound to identify and characterize a variety of DCIS lesions. Sonography may provide additional prognostic information beyond that obtained with mammography, and ultrasound provides an alternative method for biopsying and localizing lesions containing DCIS.

Acknowledgments

The author thanks Joanne VanderDoes, RDMS, and Shannon Boswell, RDMS, for their technical support and assistance in manuscript preparation. She also thanks her colleagues Drs. Steven Adler, Grady Hartzog, Dawna Kramer, Marie Lee, Gail Morgan, and Alexi Phinney for sharing their clinical experiences and cases.

References

[1] Page DL, Dupont WD, Rogers LW, et al. Continued local recurrence of carcinoma 15–25 years after a diagnosis of low grade ductal carcinoma in situ of the breast treated only with biopsy. Cancer 1995;76(7):1197–200.
[2] Page DL, Simpson JF. Ductal carcinoma in situ—the focus for prevention, screening, and breast conservation in breast cancer. N Engl J Med 1999;340(19):1499–500.
[3] Morrow M, Harris J. Ductal carcinoma in situ and microinvasive carcinoma. In: Harris JR, Lippman ME, Morrow M, et al, editors. Diseases of the breast. 3rd edition. Philadelphia: Lippincott Williams and Wilkins; 2005. p. 521–37.
[4] Frykberg E, Bland K. Current concepts on the biology and management of in situ (tis, stage 0) breast carcinoma. In: Bland KI, Copeland III EM, editors. The breast. 2nd edition. Philadelphia: W.B. Saunders; 1998. p. 1012–43.
[5] Tavassoli FA. Ductal intraepithelial neoplasia. In: Tavassoli FA, editor. Pathology of the breast. 2nd edition. Stamford (CT): Appleton and Lange; 1999. p. 205–323.
[6] Patchefsky AS, Shaber GS, Schwartz GF, et al. The pathology of breast cancer detected by mass population screening. Cancer 1977;40(4):1659–70.
[7] Stomper PC, Margolin FR. Ductal carcinoma in situ: the mammographer's perspective. AJR Am J Roentgenol 1994;162(3):585–91.
[8] Moskowitz M, Pemmaraju S, Fidler JA, et al. On the diagnosis of minimal breast cancer in a screenee population. Cancer 1976;37(5):2543–52.

[9] Tot T, Tabar L, Dean PB. Normal breast tissue or fibrocystic change?. In: Tot T, Tabar L, Dean PB, editors. Practical breast pathology. New York: Thieme; 2002. p. 1–23.

[10] Tot T, Tabar L, Dean PB. Hyperplastic changes with and without atypia. In: Tot T, Tabar L, Dean PB, editors. Practical breast pathology. New York: Thieme; 2002. p. 35–43.

[11] Tot T, Tabar L, Dean PB. Ductal carcinoma in situ (DCIS). In: Tot T, Tabar L, Dean PB, editors. Practical breast pathology. New York: Thieme; 2002. p. 45–62.

[12] Tavassoli FA. Normal development and anomalies. In: Tavassoli FA, editor. Pathology of the breast. Stamford (CT): Appleton and Lange; 1999. p. 1–25.

[13] Styblo TM, Wood WC. Traditional prognostic factors for breast cancer. In: Bland KI, Copeland III EM, editors. The breast. 2nd edition. Philadelphia: W.B. Saunders; 1998. p. 419–34.

[14] Holland R, Hendriks JH, Vebeek AL, et al. Extent, distribution, and mammographic/histological correlations of breast ductal carcinoma in situ. Lancet 1990;335(8688):519–22.

[15] Silverstein MJ, Waisman JR, Gamagami P, et al. Intraductal carcinoma of the breast (208 cases). Clinical factors influencing treatment choice. Cancer 1990;66(1):102–8.

[16] Fisher B, Costantino J, Redmond C, et al. Lumpectomy compared with lumpectomy and radiation therapy for the treatment of intraductal breast cancer. N Engl J Med 1993;328(22):1581–6.

[17] Fisher ER, Costantino J, Fisher B, et al. Pathologic findings from the National Surgical Adjuvant Breast Project (NSABP) Protocol B-17. Intraductal carcinoma (ductal carcinoma in situ). The National Surgical Adjuvant Breast and Bowel Project Collaborating Investigators. Cancer 1995;75(6):1310–9.

[18] Lagios MD, Page DL. Pathology of malignant lesions. In: Bland KI, Copeland III EM, editors. The breast. 2nd edition. Philadelphia: W.B. Saunders; 1998. p. 261–83.

[19] Ikeda DM, Andersson I. Ductal carcinoma in situ: atypical mammographic appearances. Radiology 1989;172(3):661–6.

[20] Stomper PC, Connolly JL, Meyer JE, et al. Clinically occult ductal carcinoma in situ detected with mammography: analysis of 100 cases with radiologic-pathologic correlation. Radiology 1989;172(1):235–41.

[21] Dershaw DD, Abramson A, Kinne DW. Ductal carcinoma in situ: mammographic findings and clinical implications. Radiology 1989;170(2):411–5.

[22] Huynh PT, Parellada JA, de Paredes ES, et al. Dilated duct pattern at mammography. Radiology 1997;204(1):137–41.

[23] Mitnick JS, Roses DF, Harris MN, et al. Circumscribed intraductal carcinoma of the breast. Radiology 1989;170(2):423–5.

[24] Vora SA, Wazer DE, Homer MJ. Management of microcalcifications that develop at the lumpectomy site after breast conserving therapy. Radiology 1997;203(3):667–71.

[25] Fu KL, Fu YS, Lopez JK, et al. Noninvasive carcinoma. In: Bassett LW, Jackson VP, Fu KL, et al, editors. Diagnosis of diseases of the breast. 2nd edition. Philadelphia: Elsevier; 2005. p. 467–81.

[26] Bassett LW. Mammographic analysis of calcifications. Radiol Clin North Am 1992;30(1):93–105.

[27] Meyer JE, Eberlein TJ, Stomper PC, et al. Biopsy of occult breast lesions. Analysis of 1261 abnormalities. JAMA 1990;263(17):2341–3.

[28] Gershon-Cohen J, Berger SM. Breast cancer with microcalcifications: diagnostic difficulties. Radiology 1966;87(4):613–22.

[29] Gershon-Cohen J, Yiu LS, Berger SM. The diagnostic importance of calcareous patterns in roentgenography of breast cancer. Am J Roentgenol Radium Ther Nucl Med 1962;88:1117–25.

[30] Sickles EA. Breast calcifications: mammographic evaluation. Radiology 1986;160(2):289–93.

[31] Roses DF, Harris MN, Gorstein F, et al. Biopsy for microcalcification detected by mammography. Surgery 1980;87(3):248–52.

[32] Murphy WA, DeSchryver-Kecskemeti K. Isolated clustered microcalcifications in the breast: radiologic-pathologic correlation. Radiology 1978;127(2):335–41.

[33] Colbassani HJ Jr, Feller WF, Cigtay OS, et al. Mammographic and pathologic correlation of microcalcification in disease of the breast. Surg Gynecol Obstet 1982;155(5):689–96.

[34] Hilton SV, Leopold GR, Olson LK, et al. Real-time breast sonography: application in 300 consecutive patients. AJR Am J Roentgenol 1986;147(3):479–86.

[35] Buchberger W, DeKoekkoek-Doll P, et al. Incidental findings on sonography of the breast: clinical significance and diagnostic workup. AJR Am J Roentgenol 1999;173(4):921–7.

[36] Ahmed A. Calcification in human breast carcinomas: ultrastructural observations. J Pathol 1975;117(4):247–51.

[37] Asch T, Frey C. Radiographic appearance of mammary duct ectasia with calcification. N Engl J Med 1962;266:86–7.

[38] Baker JA, Kornguth PJ, Soo MS, et al. Sonography of solid breast lesions: observer variability of lesion description and assessment. AJR Am J Roentgenol 1999;172(6):1621–5.

[39] Bird RE. Critical pathways in analyzing breast calcifications. Radiographics 1995;15(4):928–34.

[40] Evans WP III, Starr AL, Bennos ES. Comparison of the relative incidence of impalpable invasive breast carcinoma and ductal carcinoma in situ in cancers detected in patients older and younger than 50 years of age. Radiology 1997;204(2):489–91.

[41] Inoue T, Tamaki Y, Sato Y, et al. Three-dimensional ultrasound imaging of breast cancer by a real-time intraoperative navigation system. Breast Cancer 2005;12(2):122-9.

[42] Meyberg-Solomayer GC, Kraemer B, Bergmann A, et al. Does 3-D sonography bring any advantage to noninvasive breast diagnostics? Ultrasound Med Biol 2004;30(5):583-9.

[43] Fewins HE, Whitehouse GH, Leinster SJ. The spontaneous disappearance of breast calcification. Clin Radiol 1988;39(3):257-61.

[44] Goergen SK, Evans J, Cohen GP, et al. Characteristics of breast carcinomas missed by screening radiologists. Radiology 1997;204(1):131-5.

[45] Jackson VP. The current role of ultrasonography in breast imaging. Radiol Clin North Am 1995;33(6):1161-70.

[46] Sickles E. Sonographic detectability of breast calcifications. Proceedings of the Society of Photo-optical Instrumentation Engineers 1983;419:913-8.

[47] Mendelson EB, Baum JK, Berg WA, et al. Breast imaging and reporting data system ultrasound: calcifications. In: D'Orsi CJ, Bassett LW, Berg WA, et al, editors. American College of Radiology BI-RADS breast imaging and reporting data system. 4th edition. Reston (VA): American College of Radiology; 2003. p. 55-8.

[48] Yang WT, Suen M, Ahuja A, et al. In vivo demonstration of microcalcification in breast cancer using high resolution ultrasound. Br J Radiol 1997;70(835):685-90.

[49] Hashimoto BE, Kramer DJ, Picozzi VJ. High detection rate of breast ductal carcinoma in situ calcifications on mammographically directed high-resolution sonography. J Ultrasound Med 2001;20(5):501-8.

[50] Gufler H, Buitrago-Tellez CH, Madjar H, et al. Ultrasound demonstration of mammographically detected microcalcifications. Acta Radiol 2000;41(3):217-21.

[51] Moon WK, Im JG, Koh YH, et al. US of mammographically detected clustered microcalcifications. Radiology 2000;217(3):849-54.

[52] Chen SC, Cheung YC, Lo YF, et al. Sonographic differentiation of invasive and intraductal carcinomas of the breast. Br J Radiol 2003;76(909):600-4.

[53] Moon WK, Myung JS, Lee YJ, et al. US of ductal carcinoma in situ. Radiographics 2002;22(2):269-81.

[54] Satake H, Shimamoto K, Sawaki A, et al. Role of ultrasonography in the detection of intraductal spread of breast cancer: correlation with pathologic findings, mammography and MR imaging. Eur Radiol 2000;10(11):1726-32.

[55] Schoonjans JM, Brem RF. Sonographic appearance of ductal carcinoma in situ diagnosed with ultrasonographically guided large core needle biopsy: correlation with mammographic and pathologic findings. J Ultrasound Med 2000;19(7):449-57.

[56] Dogan BE, Ceyhan K, Tukel S, et al. Ductal dilatation as the manifesting sign of invasive ductal carcinoma. J Ultrasound Med 2005;24(10):1413-7.

[57] Cho N, Moon WK, Chung SY, et al. Ductographic findings of breast cancer. Korean J Radiol 2005;6(1):31-6.

[58] Wright B, Shumak R. Part II. Medical imaging of ductal carcinoma in situ. Curr Probl Cancer 2000;24(3):112-24.

[59] Hashimoto BE, Bauermeister D. Masses poorly identified mammographically: palpable masses—case 195. In: Breast imaging: a correlative atlas. New York: Thieme; 2003. p. 495-6.

[60] Stavros AT. Ultrasound of solid breast nodules: distinguishing benign from malignant. In: Breast ultrasound. Philadelphia: Lippincott, Williams and Wilkins; 2004. p. 445-527.

[61] Stavros AT. Malignant solid breast nodules: specific types. In: Breast ultrasound. Philadelphia: Lippincott Williams and Wilkins; 2004. p. 603.

[62] Stavros AT. Sonographic evaluation of breast cysts. In: Breast ultrasound. Philadelphia: Lippincott Williams and Wilkins; 2004. p. 276-350.

[63] Rickard MT. Ultrasound of malignant breast microcalcifications: role in evaluation and guided procedures. Australas Radiol 1996;40(1):26-31.

[64] Kaufman CS, Jacobson L, Bachman B, et al. Intraoperative ultrasonography guidance is accurate and efficient according to results in 100 breast cancer patients. Am J Surg 2003;186(4):378-82.

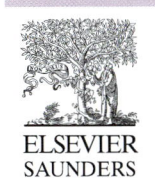

ULTRASOUND CLINICS

Sonography of Invasive Lobular Carcinoma

Gary J. Whitman, MD[a,*], Phan T. Huynh, MD[b], Parul Patel, MS[c], Joella Wilson, BS[d], Angelica Cantu[e], Savitri Krishnamurthy, MD[f]

- Pathology
- Clinical presentation
- Mammography
- MR imaging
- Sonography
- Multifocal and multicentric disease
- Axillary lymph node metastases
- Combined mammography, sonography, and MR imaging
- Summary
- Acknowledgments
- References

Invasive lobular carcinoma (ILC) is the second most common type of breast cancer, after invasive ductal carcinoma (IDC). ILC accounts for 5% to 14% of all breast cancers [1–3]. ILC is often difficult to detect due to its infiltrative pattern, with poorly defined masses on mammography and subtle thickening on physical examination. Ultrasound can be helpful in demonstrating evidence of ILC. This article reviews the histopathologic and imaging features of ILC, with an emphasis on sonography.

Pathology

ILC is composed of small round cells with scant cytoplasm and a bland appearance [2]. On histopathology, ILC tends to infiltrate in a single-file pattern, frequently encircling ducts and lobules in a targetoid manner. Usually, ILC forms a mass that can be identified on clinical examination or mammography (Fig. 1). ILC may not be detected on physical examination or mammography. In some of these cases, vague thickening may be noted retrospectively on clinical examination, or architectural distortion may be identified retrospectively on mammography. In addition, ILC has a substantially increased propensity for multifocality, multicentricity, and bilaterality compared with IDC [1,2,4–9]. Thus, breast conservation therapy may be challenging in ILC [1–3].

ILC comprises several subtypes, including the classic, alveolar, trabecular, solid, tubulo-lobular, signet ring, and pleomorphic forms [10]. About one half of all ILC cases are classified as classic. Classic ILC is the subtype most likely to present as a spiculated mass or a region of architectural distortion on mammography [11]. On gross pathology,

---

[a] Department of Diagnostic Radiology, The University of Texas M. D. Anderson Cancer Center, PO Box 301439, Unit 1350, Houston, TX 77230, USA
[b] Women's Center, St. Luke's Episcopal Hospital, 6624 Fannin, Houston, TX 77030, USA
[c] SUNY Upstate Medical University, 750 East Adams Street, Syracuse, NY 13210-2375, USA
[d] The University of Kansas School of Medicine, Mail Stop 1049, 3901 Rainbow Boulevard, Kansas City, KS 66160, USA
[e] Texas A&M University, College Station, 1244 Navajo Road, Donna, TX 78537, USA
[f] Department of Pathology, The University of Texas M. D. Anderson Cancer Center, 1515 Holcombe Boulevard, Unit 53, Houston, TX 77030, USA
* Corresponding author.
E-mail address: gwhitman@di.mdacc.tmc.edu (G.J. Whitman).

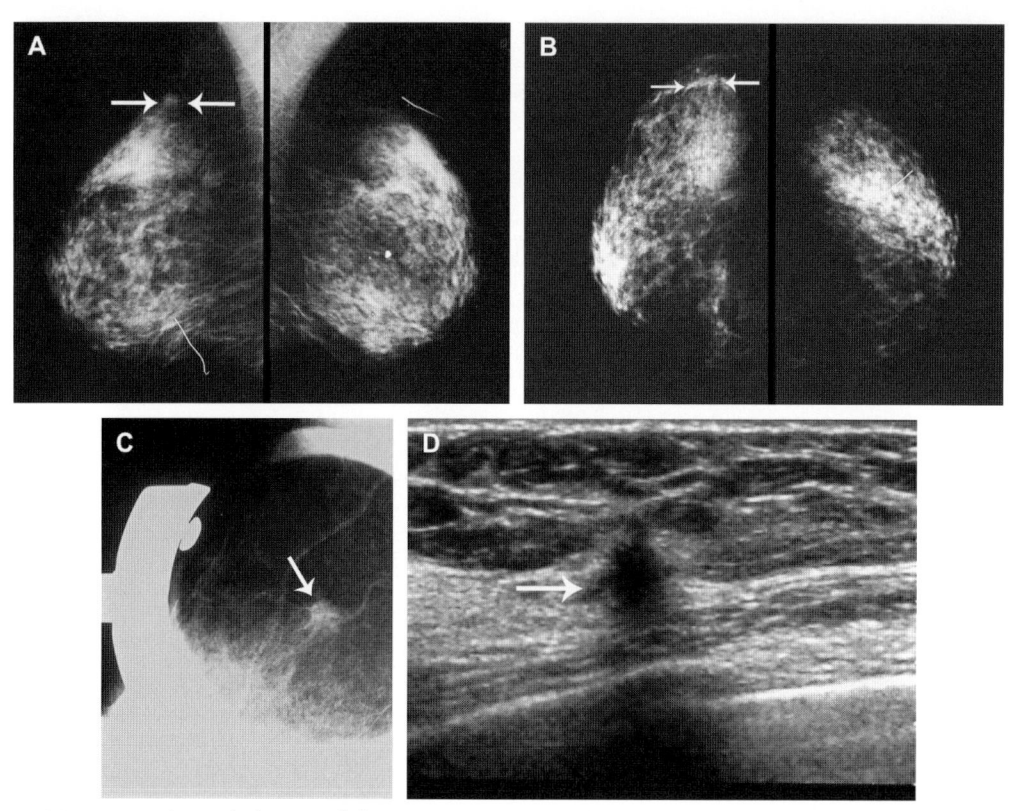

Fig. 1. Mammography and ultrasound demonstrate a mass in the upper outer left breast. Linear radiopaque markers denote the sites of prior benign excisional biopsies in both breasts. (*A*) A mass is noted in the posterior upper outer left breast on the mediolateral oblique mammogram (*arrows*). (*B*) The mass (*arrows*) is also seen on the craniocaudal view. (*C*) On spot compression mammography, a spiculated mass is noted (*arrow*). (*D*) Sonography shows a hypoechoic, ill-defined mass (*arrow*) that is taller than it is wide. Pathology revealed pleomorphic ILC.

classic ILC is usually noted as a firm to hard tumor with irregular borders [12]. On microscopic evaluation, classic ILC is characterized by thread-like strands of tumor cells loosely arranged in fibrous stroma [12]. The classic type of ILC is more commonly associated with lobular carcinoma in situ (LCIS) and atypical lobular hyperplasia than the other subtypes [13]. In a study of 62 cases of ILC, Selinko and colleagues [13] noted that 70% (28/40) of classic ILCs were associated with atypical lobular hyperplasia and LCIS.

Alveolar ILC is characterized as clusters of at least 20 cells [12]. Trabecular ILC has prominent bands two or more cells broad [12]. The solid subtype is characterized by large sheets of uniform, small cells. In signet ring ILC (Fig. 2), greater than 90% of the cells have cytoplasmic, sialomucin-filled vacuoles [11]. Pleomorphic ILC demonstrates abundant, eosinophilic cytoplasm and apocrine differentiation [12]. The mixed type demonstrates features of ILC and IDC.

Compared with IDC, ILC is associated with a higher rate of hormone receptor expression and a lower rate of cellular proliferation [3]. Despite these favorable prognostic characteristics, the recurrence and survival rates for patients who have ILC are similar to those for patients who have IDC, based on stage at the time of diagnosis. The most important determinants of prognosis for women who have ILC are the size of the primary tumor and the regional lymph node status [12].

Clinical presentation

ILC is notorious for presenting subtle findings on clinical examination. Often, ILC does not form a distinct mass that may be identified by palpation. ILC may present with skin retraction and thickening, often involving the nipple [14]. Once discovered, ILCs are usually slightly larger than IDCs. ILC is more frequently multifocal and multicentric than IDC.

ILC has an unusual pattern of distant metastases. ILC metastasizes via lymphatic or hematogenous dissemination [12]. ILC may metastasize to the peritoneum (Fig. 3), ovaries, gastric mucosa,

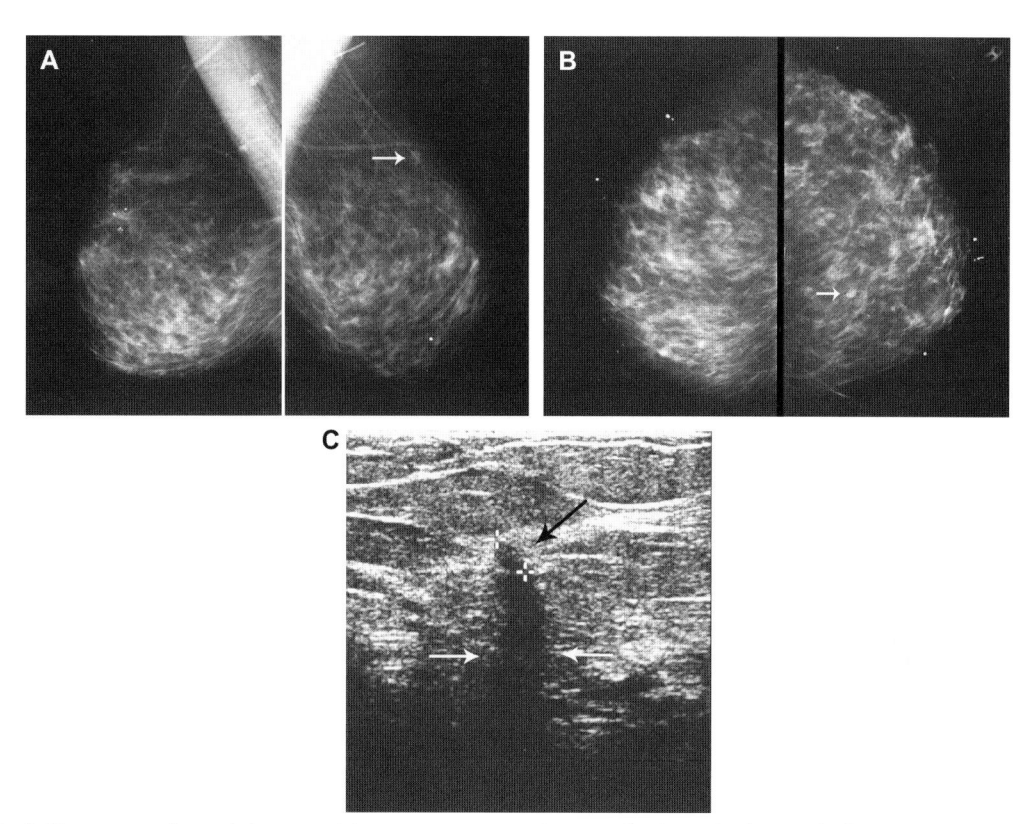

Fig. 2. Mammography and ultrasound demonstrate a new circumscribed mass in the 1 o'clock position of the right breast. (*A*) On the mediolateral oblique mammogram, the mass (*arrow*) is oval and well defined. (*B*) The mass (*arrow*) is well defined on the craniocaudal view. (*C*) On sonography, an oval hypoechoic mass (*calipers, black arrow*) is seen, with posterior acoustic shadowing (*white arrows*). Pathology revealed signet ring ILC.

endometrium, and the meninges. Although lung and brain metastases are more common in patients who have IDC, bone metastases are more common in women who have ILC [3]. It has been suggested that the loss of the cell–cell adhesion molecule E-cadherin is responsible for decreased adhesiveness in ILC tumor cells, thus facilitating metastases to locations such as the peritoneum and accounting for the increased likelihood of bilaterality, multifocality, and multicentricity [3].

Mammography

ILC often presents a diagnostic challenge on mammography. Mammography is associated with a high false-negative rate in the detection of ILC, likely due to ILC's tendency to present as an indistinct mass with a density similar to that of the adjacent fibroglandular tissues and without a desmoplastic reaction. In the series by Krecke and Gisvold [1], the rate of false-negative findings on initial mammographic interpretations was 19%. In 46% of the mammograms with false-negative initial interpretations, no evidence of malignancy was identified in retrospect. Another factor contributing to false-negative mammography in patients who have ILC is that ILC is rarely associated with suspicious calcifications. IDC, on the other hand, is often identified

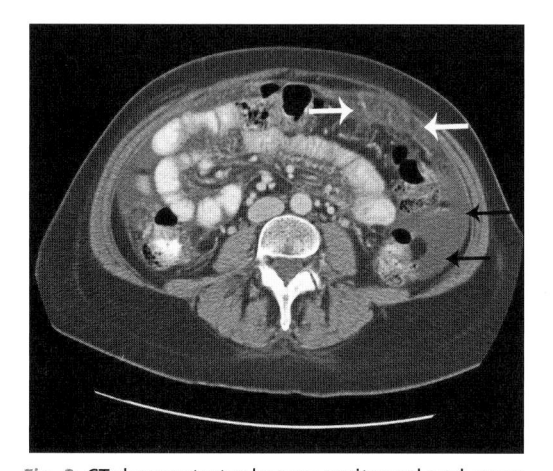

Fig. 3. CT demonstrates known peritoneal and omental metastases in a 52-year-old woman who has a history of ILC. Nodularity is noted in the omentum (*white arrows*), and a moderate amount of ascites is identified (*black arrows*).

on mammography as a suspicious cluster of microcalcifications, with or without an associated mass. In the series by Krecke and Gisvold, suspicious calcifications prompted biopsy in 1% of the patients who had ILC. In that series, 10% of the ILCs had mammographically detectable calcifications [1].

Cornford and colleagues [4] noted that calcifications were identified less frequently in ILC compared with IDC. In the study by Cornford and colleagues, 86 biopsy-proven cases of ILC were compared with 86 biopsy-proven cases of IDC, matched for age, size, and stage. The authors noted that ILC was often indistinguishable from IDC on mammography. For IDC and ILC, the most common finding on mammography was a spiculated mass. Spiculated masses were identified in 69% of the ILCs and in 63% of the IDCs. ILC was more likely than IDC to be associated with a mammographic finding seen only on one view. In seven patients (8%) who had ILC, the mammographic abnormality was demonstrated on only one view.

Newstead and colleagues [6] analyzed the mammographic features of 316 cases of breast carcinoma. Mammography demonstrated malignant calcifications in 110 of 229 cases (47%) of IDC and in none of 37 cases of ILC. Asymmetric densities (Fig. 4) and architectural distortion were the predominant findings in 21 of 37 (57%) cases of ILC. Of the 34 mammographically detectable ILC lesions, 29 (85%) were less dense or equally dense as the normal fibroglandular tissue. Eleven (32%) of the 34 mammographically detectable ILCs were perceived initially in only one mammographic view. ILC was usually best identified on the craniocaudal views, whereas IDC was usually best seen on the mediolateral oblique views.

Le Gal and colleagues [15] reviewed the mammograms in 6009 cases of breast cancer. Four hundred fifty-five (7.6%) of the tumors were ILCs. The authors compared the mammographic features of the ILC and the IDC cases. ILC presented less frequently than IDC as a round mass. ILC was identified more frequently as a spiculated mass (28% versus 23%) or as a region of architectural distortion (18% versus 6%) compared with IDC. Microcalcifications were less common in ILC (24% versus 41%) than in IDC. Retraction of the skin (25% versus 21%) and the nipple (26% versus 17%) was more common in ILC than in IDC. When magnification views were obtained, they were considered helpful in diagnosing half of the cases of ILC and 75% of the cases of IDC [15].

Decreased breast size secondary to ILC (Fig. 5) has been reported. Decreased breast size may be identified on clinical examination or on mammography (Fig. 6). Harvey and colleagues [16] retrospectively evaluated the mammograms in 30 patients who had ILC and noted an ipsilateral decrease in mammographic size in five patients (17%). In the report by Harvey and colleagues, the patients who had an ipsilateral decrease in breast size had more subtle mammographic findings (Fig. 7) than the patients who had no decrease in breast size. None of the patients who had a decrease in mammographic size had masses on mammography, whereas 13 of the 25 patients (52%) who had no change in mammographic size had mammographic masses.

In the future, computer-assisted detection devices are likely to help radiologists in finding ILC on mammography. In a retrospective study, the sensitivity of computer-assisted detection devices was 91% (86/94) for all ILCs and 94% (58/62) for all pure ILCs [17]. Contralateral breast cancer and multicentric and multifocal disease are more common in ILC than in IDC [18]. Thus, sonography and MR imaging may be helpful in identifying additional sites of disease in women who have known or suspected ILC. MR imaging is useful for evaluating the contralateral breast and for identifying additional foci of ILC in the ipsilateral breast.

MR imaging

Dynamic contrast-enhanced MR imaging is a valuable tool in evaluating patients who have known or suspected ILC. MR imaging combines assessment of architectural features with analysis of tumor vascularity. MR imaging is particularly helpful in demonstrating multifocal and multicentric disease. MR imaging has been shown to be efficacious in preoperative planning to assess if breast conservation surgery is appropriate.

Breast MR imaging has a sensitivity of 94% to 100% and a specificity of 37% to 97% for detection of invasive breast cancer. Bartella and colleagues [19] retrospectively reviewed the MR imaging findings in 68 nonpalpable, mammographically occult cancers in 57 women. Histopathology demonstrated IDC in 65% (44/68), mixed invasive ductal and lobular carcinoma in 19% (13/68), and ILC in 16% (11/68). On MR imaging, 57% (25/44) of IDCs and 73% (8/11) of ILCs were evident as nonmass lesions. Forty-three percent (19/44) of IDCs and 27% (3/11) of ILCs were identified as mass lesions.

Weinstein and colleagues [20] evaluated the MR imaging findings in 31 women diagnosed with pure ILC. In 7 of 18 women who did not undergo excisional biopsy before the MR imaging, MR imaging demonstrated a more extensive tumor burden compared with mammography and sonography or revealed a primary tumor that was not identified on mammography or sonography. In 9

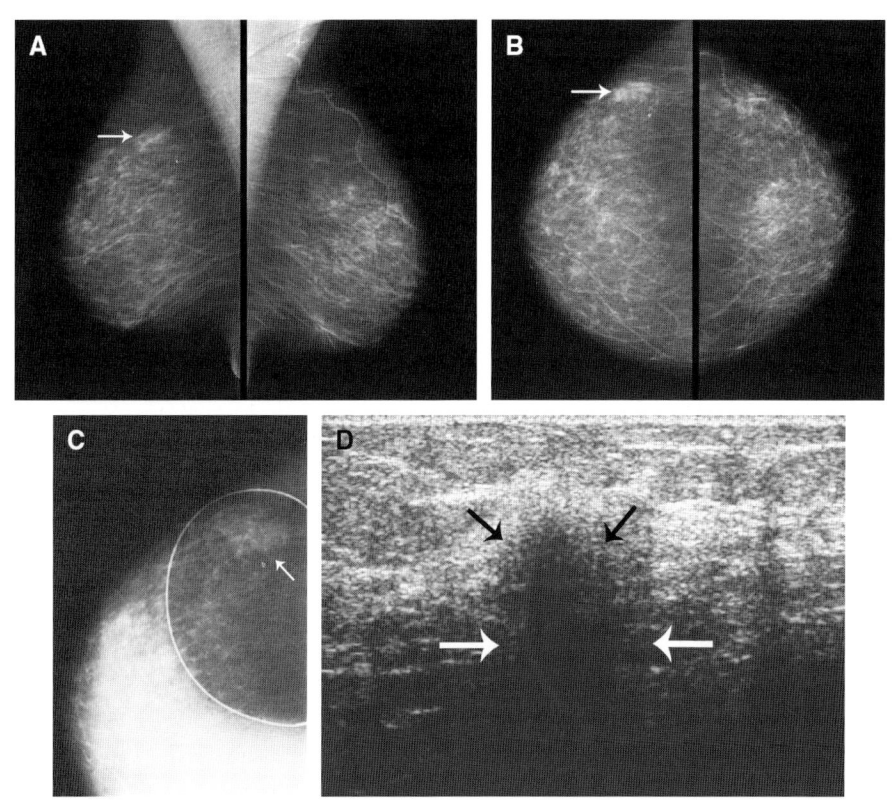

Fig. 4. Mammography and ultrasound demonstrate a focal asymmetry in the left breast in a 72-year-old woman. (*A*) The mediolateral oblique mammogram shows focal asymmetry (*arrow*) in the posterior upper left breast. (*B*) Focal asymmetry (*arrow*) is noted in the outer left breast on the craniocaudal view. (*C*) On spot compression mammography, the mass (*arrow*) is less dense and less clearly defined. (*D*) On ultrasound, a hypoechoic mass (*black arrows*) is noted, along with posterior acoustic shadowing (*white arrows*). Biopsy demonstrated ILC.

of 18 women (50%), MR imaging performed equally as well as mammography and sonography. In one case, MR imaging overestimated the tumor extent, and mammography failed to demonstrate the cancer [20].

In the study by Weinstein and colleagues [20], 14 patients underwent excisional biopsy before MR imaging. Residual tumor was shown on MR imaging in 8 of 14 patients (57%), with extensive tumor noted in four patients and an additional tumor focus demonstrated in one patient. All five of these patients had negative mammographic examinations before their initial excisional biopsies. Two postoperative MR imaging studies were interpreted as equivocal for evidence of malignancy, and residual tumor was identified in both cases on re-excision. In three cases, postoperative MR imaging studies were interpreted as negative for malignancy, but microscopic tumor was noted around the seroma on re-excision. There was one false-positive MR imaging study in which suspicious contrast enhancement was noted around the seroma, but re-excision revealed no evidence of residual tumor.

Overall, in the study by Weinstein and colleagues [20], MR imaging revealed more extensive malignancy than mammography and sonography. MR imaging affected clinical management decisions in half (16/32) of the patients who had ILC. Weinstein and colleagues noted that MR imaging can play an important role in cases in which breast conservation therapy is being considered because ILC has a propensity to be multifocal in 14% to 31% of cases. The authors indicated that the inability to detect macroscopic residual disease or multifocal disease could lead to failure of breast conservation due to recurrence.

Yeh and colleagues [21] evaluated the morphology and enhancement patterns on MR imaging in 19 patients who had ILC. The authors noted that in the majority of cases, ILC was identified with MR imaging on the basis of morphologic features and contrast enhancement patterns. There were variable morphologic appearances and contrast enhancement patterns, and in some cases, ILC was difficult to distinguish from normal tissues. In some cases without a mass, the enhancement may

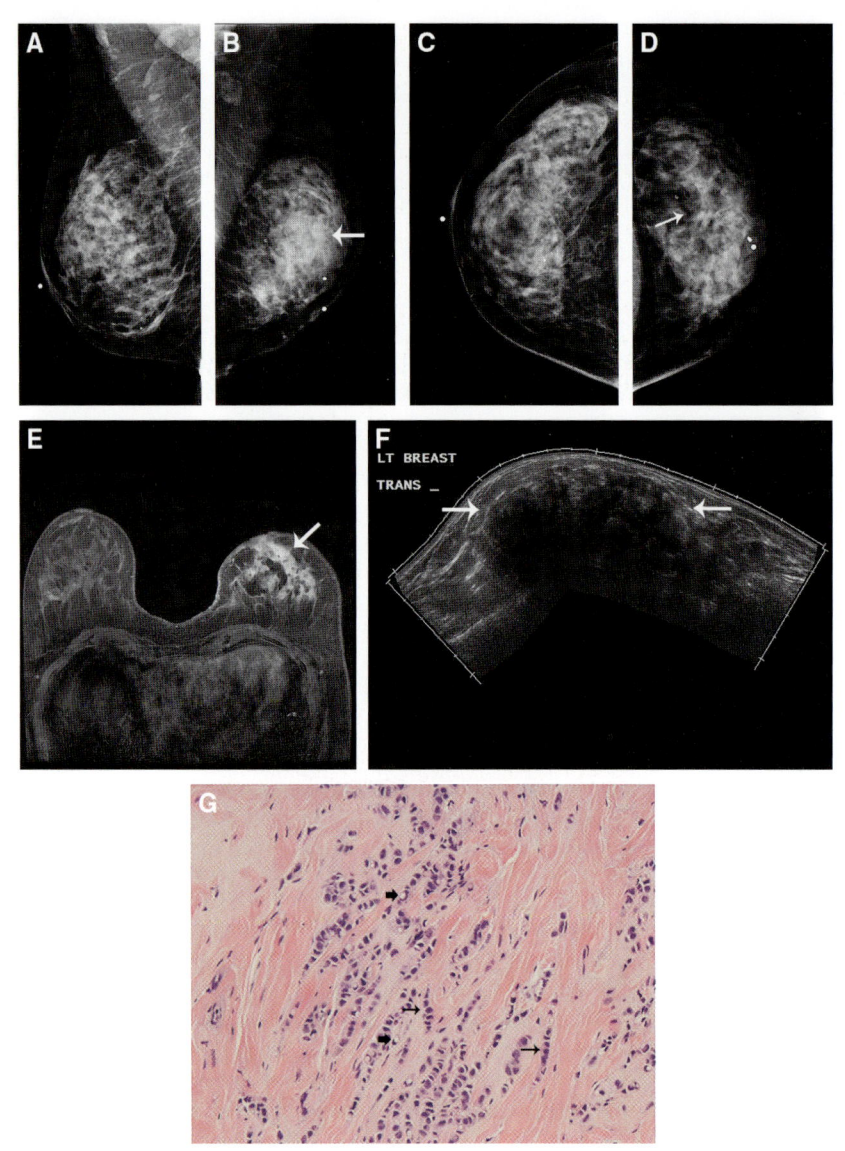

Fig. 5. Mammography, sonography, and MR imaging demonstrate decreased breast size in a 68-year-old woman. (*A*) The right mediolateral oblique mammogram is unremarkable. (*B*) The left mediolateral oblique view demonstrates that the left breast is smaller than the right breast, and increased density is noted in the upper left breast (*arrow*). (*C*) The right craniocaudal view is unremarkable. (*D*) The left craniocaudal mammogram shows that the left breast is smaller than the right breast. Architectural distortion (*arrow*) is noted in the left breast. (*E*) Axial postcontrast MR imaging shows diffuse enhancement in the left breast (*arrow*), which is smaller than the right breast. (*F*) Transverse extended field-of-view sonogram shows a large hypoechoic mass (*arrows*) with posterior shadowing. (*G*) Photomicrograph shows evidence of ILC with discohesive tumor cells of intermediate grade arranged predominantly in linear cords (*long arrows*) with a few interspersed signet ring cells (*short arrows*) (hematoxylin-eosin, original magnification ×20).

be similar to that of normal tissues in premenopausal women or in postmenopausal women on hormone replacement therapy. The authors noted that these findings may be due to the insidious infiltration of ILC without an associated desmoplastic reaction.

Sonography may be helpful in clarifying subtle or equivocal mammographic or MR imaging findings and in guiding biopsies of suspicious masses and regions of architectural distortion (Fig. 8). If a suspicious lesion is identified on MR imaging, sonography should be performed, and if the targeted

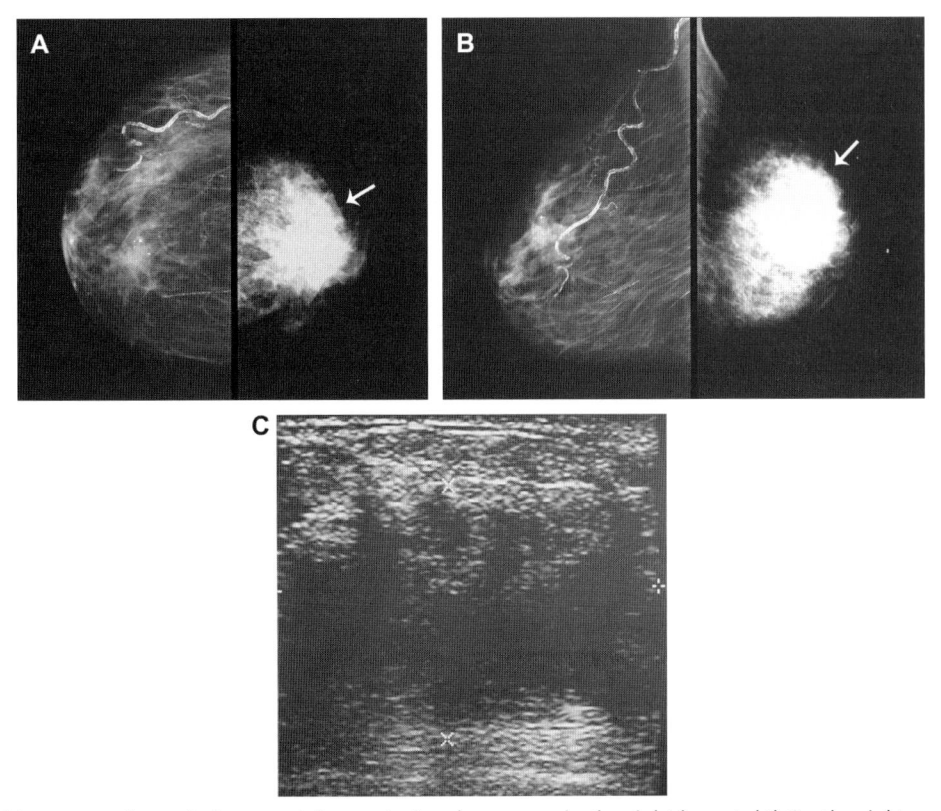

Fig. 6. Mammography and ultrasound demonstrate a large mass in the right breast. (*A*) On the right mediolateral oblique mammogram, a large, high-density, ill-defined mass occupies the entire right breast (*arrow*). (*B*) On the right craniocaudal mammogram, the large mass is noted (*arrow*). The right breast is smaller than the left breast. (*C*) On ultrasound, there is an ill-defined, hypoechoic mass (*calipers*), representing biopsy-proven ILC.

lesion is demonstrated on sonography, ultrasound-guided biopsy should be performed rather than MR imaging–guided biopsy because ultrasound guidance is cheaper, quicker, and more comfortable for the patient.

Sonography

Over the last decade, sonography had become an integral component of most breast imaging practices. Ultrasound is commonly used to determine if a mammographic or a palpable abnormality (Fig. 9) is a real mass. If ultrasound reveals a suspicious abnormality, then biopsy with sonographic guidance should be performed.

Chapellier and colleagues [22] described the ultrasound findings in 102 cases of ILC. In five cases, proven ILCs were not identified on sonography. In the remaining 97 cases identified on ultrasound, irregular, heterogeneous, hypoechoic masses were noted in 94 cases, and there was associated posterior acoustic shadowing in 87 cases. In three cases, posterior acoustic shadowing was the only finding on sonography. All five of the palpable ILCs not identified on mammography were demonstrated on sonography. In the series by Chapellier and colleagues, sonography successfully visualized 19 of 22 ILCs that were less than 1 cm in size.

Cawson and colleagues [23] examined the clinical, mammographic, sonographic, and histopathologic features of 62 ILCs detected on screening mammography. Comparison was made to 60 screen-detected IDCs. The sensitivity of sonography for demonstrating ILC in the lesions examined was 88% (36/41). Four ILCs were not detected on sonography, and one ILC was misclassified as a benign lesion. The mean diameter of the ILCs identified on ultrasound was 17.6 mm. Fifteen out of 62 ILCs in the series were 1 cm or less in diameter. Twelve of these 15 cases were examined with sonography, and ultrasound demonstrated ILC in 11 cases.

In the series by Cawson and colleagues [23], 33 of the 37 ILCs (89%) visible on sonography had irregular, spiculated margins, and four had smooth margins. Posterior acoustic attenuation was noted in 33 out of 37 ILCs (89%). Nine of the 37 ILCs

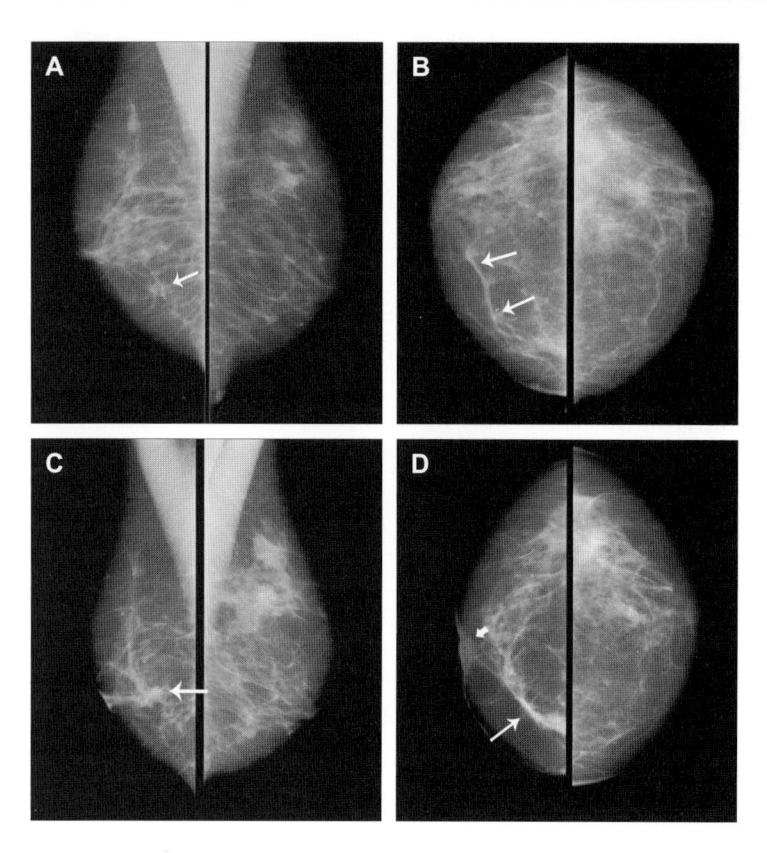

Fig. 7. Serial mammograms 1 year apart demonstrate a decrease in the size of the left breast on mammography. (*A*) Initial left mediolateral oblique mammogram demonstrates thickening (*arrows*) of the breast parenchyma. (*B*) Initial left craniocaudal mammogram shows thickening (*arrows*). (*C*) Left mediolateral oblique mammogram obtained 1 year later shows architectural distortion (*long arrow*). (*D*) Leftcraniocaudal mammogram obtained 1 year after the initial examination demonstrates distortion (*long arrow*) and nipple retraction (*short arrow*). Biopsy demonstrated ILC.

(24%) demonstrated a taller than wide shape. Sixteen of 37 (43%) ILCs were hypoechoic or isoechoic, and 21 (57%) were hyperechoic (Fig. 10) or had a significant hyperechoic component. The hyperechoic pattern may be secondary to ILC's tendency to infiltrate as rows of single cells into surrounding parenchyma and in concentric rings around normal ducts. Lesion shape and the presence of posterior acoustic shadowing were similar when the ILCs were compared with the IDCs. ILC was 9.94 times more likely to be hyperechoic than IDC, and ILC was 77% less likely to be taller than wide than IDC.

Waterman and colleagues [24] studied the sonographic features of 406 invasive breast cancers. Sixty-nine ILCs were compared with 337 tumors of other histologic differentiation (TOD), of which 272 were IDCs. Ten sonographic criteria were evaluated: shape, orientation, echogenicity, echo pattern, calcifications, margin, margin contour, lesion boundary, surrounding tissue, and posterior acoustic features. On histopathology, the ILCs were slightly larger than the TODs (mean of 26.9 mm versus 23.1 mm). On ultrasound, irregular shape was noted in 88% of the ILCs and in 67% of the TODs. The margins were indistinct in 94% of the ILCs, compared with 76% of the TODs. Posterior shadowing was observed in 84% of the ILCs and in 58% of the TODs. Irregular margin contour, hyper- or isoechoic pattern, and architectural distortion were more frequent in ILCs than in TODs. Underestimation of tumor size by ultrasound was significantly more frequent in ILCs than in TODs.

Ohta and colleagues [25] compared the sonographic features of 81 IDCs (including 26 papillotubular carcinomas, 28 solid-tubular carcinomas, and 27 scirrhous carcinomas) with 24 ILCs. The authors noted that it was difficult to distinguish ILC from scirrhous carcinoma on sonography. Scirrhous carcinomas and ILCs tended to be irregular, ill-defined tumors, with associated posterior shadowing. The authors noted that, in general, the papillotubular carcinomas and the solid-tubular carcinomas had a low frequency of malignant sonographic findings, whereas the scirrhous carcinomas and the ILCs had a high frequency of malignant findings.

In the analysis by Ohta and colleagues [25], the sensitivities of sonography for tumor detection were 88.5% for papillotubular carcinoma, 100% for solid-tubular carcinoma, 92.6% for scirrhous carcinoma, and 91.7% for ILC. The mean diameter of the two ILCs not identified on ultrasound was 8.9 cm, compared with 1.2 cm for the IDC cases. The authors noted that large ILCs may be non–mass forming on sonography.

In some cases, ILC may present on sonography as architectural distortion, with or without posterior acoustic shadowing, and without a definable mass

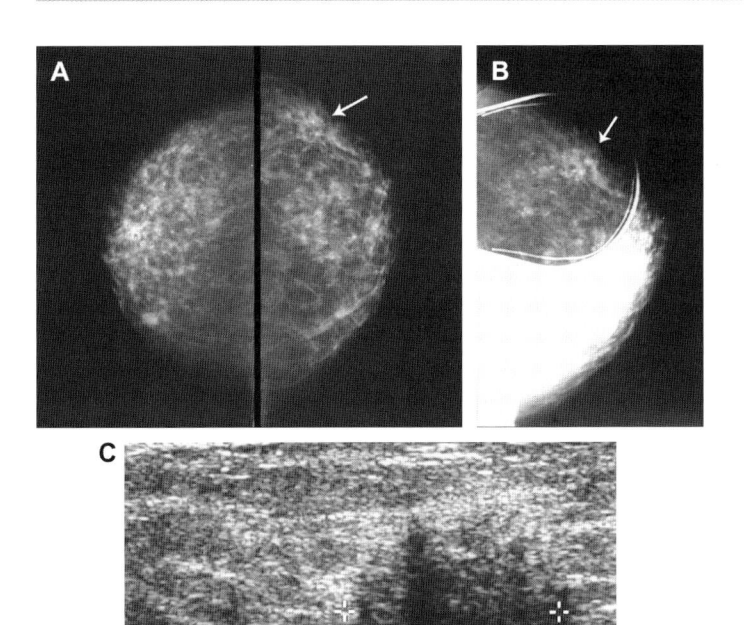

Fig. 8. Ultrasound was performed after mammography, which revealed architectural distortion. (*A*) The right craniocaudal mammogram demonstrates architectural distortion (*arrow*). (*B*) The right craniocaudal spot compression view shows persistent distortion (*arrow*). (*C*) Sonography demonstrates a hypoechoic mass (*calipers*) with posterior acoustic shadowing (*arrow*). Pathology revealed classic ILC.

(Fig. 11). Rissanen and colleagues [26] reviewed the sonographic and mammographic findings in 63 cases of pure ILC. Fifty-one of the ILCs were identified on mammography, and 49 of the ILCs were demonstrated on ultrasound. In six cases, the only positive findings on sonography were architectural distortions with posterior acoustic shadowing. In four of these cases, the mammographic correlates were asymmetric densities.

Butler and colleagues [27] reviewed the sonographic findings in 81 cases of ILC. In 49 of 81 cases (60.5%), ILC was seen as a heterogeneous, hypoechoic mass with angular or ill-defined margins and posterior acoustic shadowing. Of the remaining 32 ILCs, 12 showed focal shadowing without a discrete mass; 10 appeared as lobulated, well circumscribed masses; and 10 were not visible on sonography. In the study by Butler and colleagues, classic ILC tended to present as focal shadowing without a discrete mass, and pleomorphic ILC typically was seen as a shadowing mass. Of all the subtypes, signet ring, alveolar, and solid ILCs were most likely to be seen on ultrasound as lobulated, well circumscribed masses. In 81 cases in which the mammographic findings were subtle or invisible, sonography detected 71 ILCs (87.7%). The sensitivity of sonography for detecting ILC less than 1 cm in size was 85.7% (12/14).

Ashkar and colleagues [28] noted that the sensitivity in the detection of ILC on mammography has been reported to be as low as 65%, whereas sonography has been shown to have a higher sensitivity (88%–98%), especially when high-frequency transducers are used. Askar and colleagues emphasized that although most ILCs are hypoechoic masses with posterior shadowing and irregular or indistinct borders, small ILCs may have unusual sonographic characteristics, including a wider-than-tall shape, a hyperechoic component, and an infiltrative pattern. The authors noted that the morphology of ILC, with horizontal growth along normal tissue planes, may account for the wider-than-tall configuration.

Ashkar and colleagues [28] noted the importance of using high-frequency transducers to delineate the spiculations and microlobulations, which may be associated with small ILCs. The authors indicated that harmonic imaging can be helpful in detecting ILCs as subtle hypoechoic masses and in identifying posterior acoustic shadowing. They also noted that ILC may have a mixed hypo- and hyperechoic appearance, likely due to the tumor's pattern of growth. ILC infiltration into surrounding structures can lead to an increase in reflective surfaces, resulting in increased internal echoes on ultrasound.

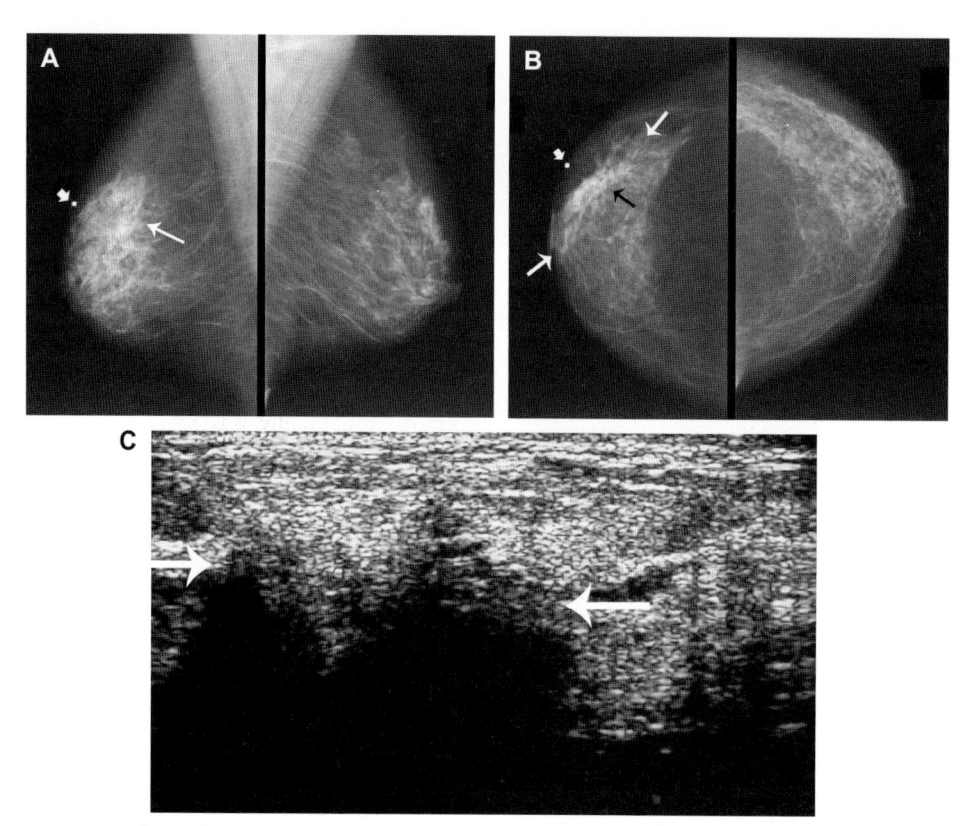

Fig. 9. Mammography and sonography were performed to evaluate a palpable abnormality in the left breast. (A) The left mediolateral oblique mammogram shows architectural distortion (*long arrow*) in the region of the palpable abnormality (*radiopaque marker, short arrow*). (B) On the left craniocaudal mammogram, distortion (*black arrow*) is noted in the region of the palpable abnormality (*radiopaque marker, short white arrow*), with extension noted medially and laterally (*long white arrows*). (C) Sonography shows a hypoechoic mass (*arrows*) with two triangular components and marked posterior acoustic shadowing. Biopsy revealed ILC. In this case, sonography provided a more accurate estimate of the size of the malignant process than mammography.

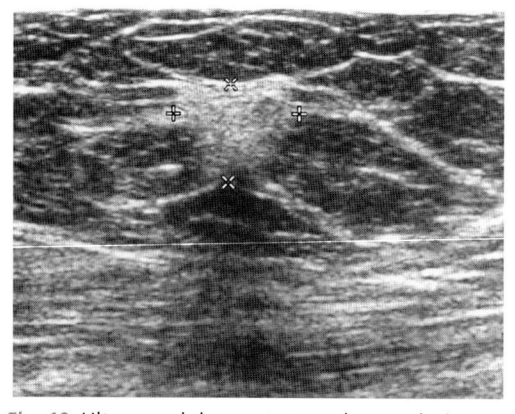

Fig. 10. Ultrasound demonstrates a hyperechoic mass in a 55-year-old woman who presented with a palpable mass. Mammography was unremarkable. On sonography, a 1-cm hyperechoic mass is noted (*calipers*). Pathology demonstrated ILC.

Selinko and colleagues [13] retrospectively reviewed 62 cases of pure ILC and found that ultrasound had a sensitivity of 98%, compared with 65% for mammography. On ultrasound, ILC was most commonly identified as a hypoechoic mass, with (58%) or without (27%) shadowing. In eight cases (13%), an infiltrative pattern, characterized as an area of altered, hypoechoic, inhomogeneous echotexture without identifiable margins and without frank shadowing, was noted. This pattern was better appreciated with extended field-of-view imaging than with conventional, small field-of-view images. The infiltrative pattern was associated with large (>5 cm) tumors that were difficult to identify on mammography and with the classic subtype of ILC. The authors noted that the infiltrative appearance was likely secondary to the pattern of tumor growth in classical and pleomorphic ILC, in which tumor-forming cords extend into the breast parenchyma in an infiltrative manner.

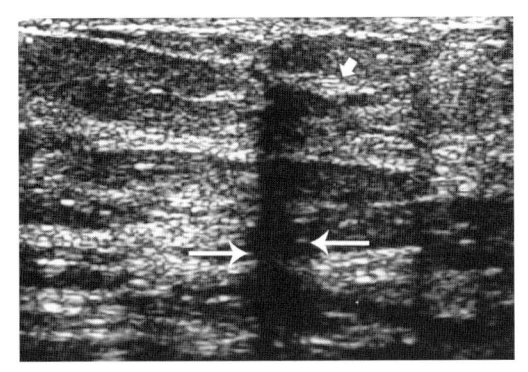

Fig. 11. A 42-year-old woman presented with thickening near the left nipple. Sonography shows a thickened Cooper's ligament (*short arrow*) and posterior acoustic shadowing (*long arrows*). Biopsy demonstrated ILC.

Shadowing only, without an associated mass, was seen in seven cases (11%). A relatively well defined mass was noted in one case (2%), and one ILC was not detected on sonography. The tumor that was not detected on ultrasound was also not seen on mammography; the missed ILC was a 0.3-cm palpable mass located near the nipple [13].

Evans and Lyons [29] reported that the vast majority of small (<1 cm) ILCs can be identified on ultrasound. In the study by Evans and Lyons, 16 cases of pure ILC with a diameter less than 1 cm were diagnosed during a 9-year study. Fourteen of 15 patients who underwent ultrasound had abnormal findings, and a definitive diagnosis of ILC was made in all 14 women with ultrasound-guided biopsy. On sonography, the most frequent finding was an ill-defined hypoechoic mass with or without posterior shadowing. In some cases, the only finding on sonography was shadowing. The authors noted that their ability to identify small ILCs was likely due to meticulous attention to the area corresponding to the region of the mammographic abnormality and the use of high-frequency transducers (up to 13 MHz).

Skaane and Skjorten [18] noted that tumors greater than 3 cm in diameter were usually underestimated by mammography and sonography. Pritt and colleagues [30] reviewed the ultrasound and

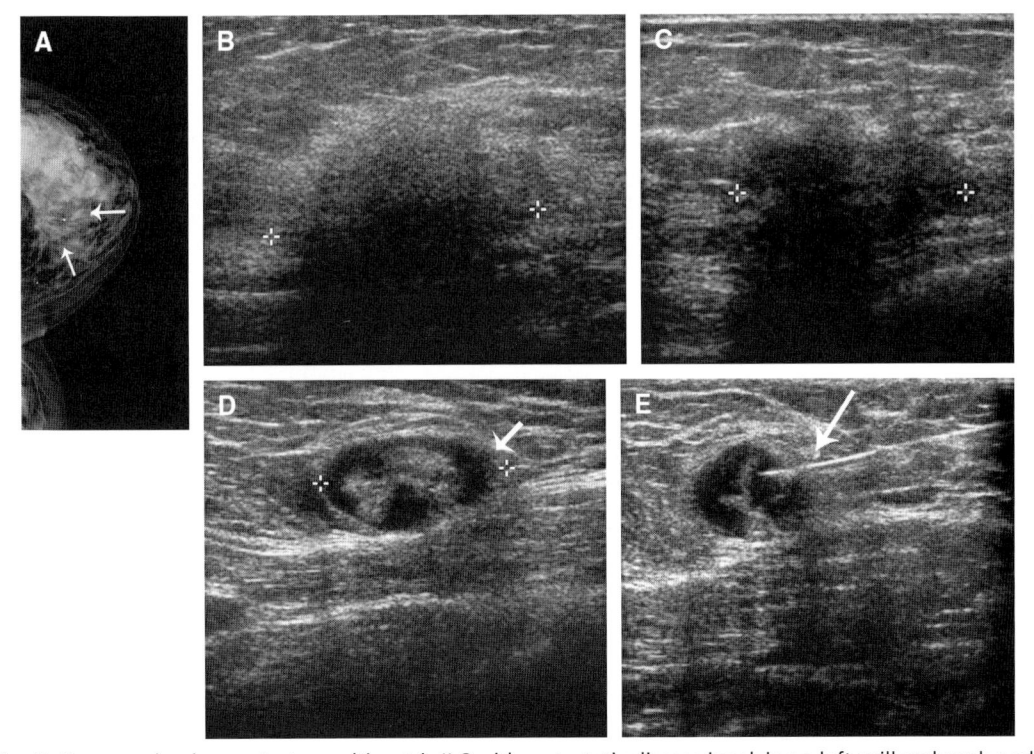

Fig. 12. Sonography demonstrates multicentric ILC with metastatic disease involving a left axillary lymph node. (*A*) On the left craniocaudal mammogram, a focus of architectural distortion is noted centrally (*arrows*). (*B*) On sonography, a hypoechoic mass (*calipers*) is seen at the 12 o'clock position, with posterior acoustic shadowing. (*C*) Ultrasound shows a second hypoechoic mass at the 3 o'clock position in the left breast (*calipers*). The mass at the 3 o'clock position was not visible on mammography. Ultrasound-guided core needle biopsy of the masses at the 12 o'clock and 3 o'clock positions revealed ILC. (*D*) Sonography shows a left axillary lymph node (*calipers*) with cortical thickening (*arrow*). (*E*) Ultrasound-guided FNA of the left axillary lymph node demonstrates the needle (*arrow*) in the region of cortical thickening. Cytology showed metastatic ILC.

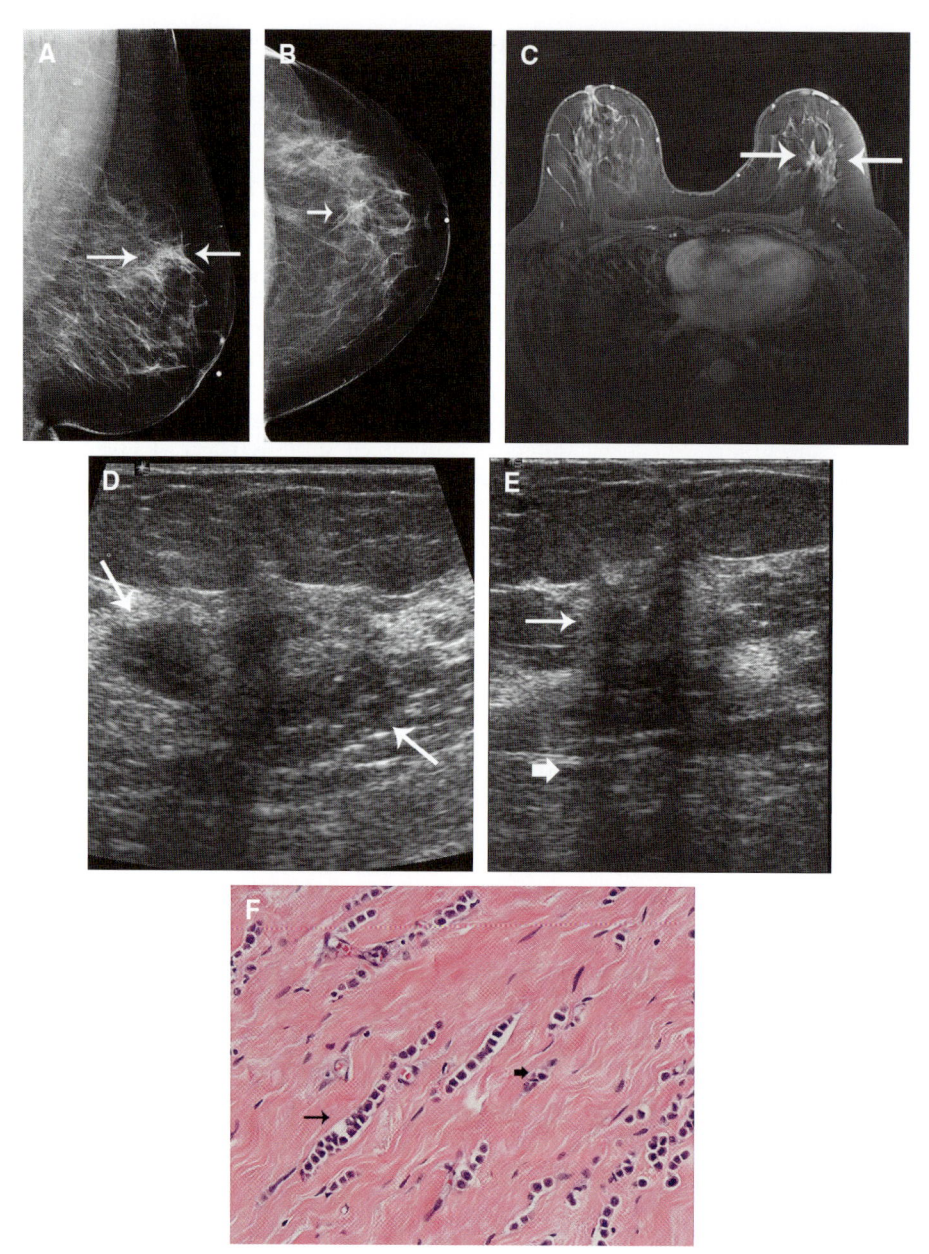

Fig. 13. Mammography, sonography, and MR imaging demonstrate ILC in the upper outer left breast in a 67-year-old woman. (*A*) The left lateromedial mammogram shows an area of architectural distortion in the upper breast (*arrows*), with an associated clip marker. The marker was placed after ultrasound-guided biopsy, which revealed ILC. (*B*) The left craniocaudal mammogram shows a central region of distortion (*arrow*) and the clip marker. (*C*) Axial postcontrast MR imaging demonstrates an irregular mass (*arrows*) with enhancement in the 12 o'clock to 1 o'clock region of the left breast. (*D*) Left breast transverse ultrasound in the 1 o'clock position demonstrates an irregular mass (*arrows*). (*E*) Longitudinal sonography in the 1 o'clock position of the left breast shows the hypoechoic mass (*large arrow*), with associated posterior acoustic shadowing (*small arrow*). (*F*) Photomicrograph shows features of classic ILC. The tumor cells with low nuclear grade features are arranged singly (*short arrow*) and linearly (*long arrow*) in a background of dense fibrosis (hematoxylin-eosin, original magnification ×20).

pathology reports in 210 invasive breast cancers, including 129 ductal, 41 lobular, and 40 mixed ductal and lobular carcinomas. Sonography consistently underestimated pathologic tumor size. The overall median difference was 3.5 mm. The median difference was 2.5 mm for IDCs, 3.0 mm for mixed carcinomas, and 7.5 mm for ILCs. The authors noted that the size difference may be large in ILC, potentially affecting staging and subsequent treatment planning.

Underestimation of ILC on ultrasound may affect surgical planning. Moore and colleagues [31] compared 47 patients with ILC who underwent breast conservation therapy with 150 patients with IDC who underwent breast conservation. Surgical margins were positive in 51% of the patients who had ILC and in 15% of the patients who had IDC. In this series, the average number of surgical procedures in the patients who had ILC was 1.64, compared with 1.15 for the patients who had IDC.

Multifocal and multicentric disease

Although sonography may underestimate the size of ILCs, whole breast sonography can be efficacious in demonstrating evidence of multifocal or multicentric disease. Wilkinson and colleagues [32] compared 102 women who had breast cancer who underwent bilateral whole breast sonography with 124 women who had breast cancer who underwent targeted breast ultrasound. Multicentric/multifocal tumors were demonstrated in 35 (34%) of the 102 study participants and in 18 (15%) of the 124 control subjects who underwent targeted breast sonography. Bilateral whole breast sonography increased the preoperative diagnosis of multiple tumors in women who had primary breast cancer, resulting in a change in management in 8% of cases. Two women had more extensive local surgery, five women were converted from local surgery to mastectomy, and one woman had an unsuspected contralateral carcinoma that was identified on sonography, resulting in a mastectomy [32].

Berg and Gilbreath [33] noted that sonography may be especially helpful in patients who have invasive lobular carcinoma because the extent of disease may be underestimated on mammography. Berg and Gilbreath performed whole breast sonography on 40 patients who had known breast cancer or in whom there was a high suspicion of malignancy. Sonography depicted 45 (94%) of 48 invasive tumor foci and 7 (44%) of 16 foci of ductal carcinoma in situ (DCIS). Mammography identified 39 (81%) of 48 invasive tumor foci and 14 (88%) of 16 foci of DCIS. Nine (14%) of 64 malignant foci were identified only on sonography, including three IDCs, two ILCs, two mixed infiltrating and intraductal cancers, and two foci of DCIS. Two (18%) of 11 foci of ILC were missed on sonography and mammography. Of 20 patients suspected of having unifocal disease on the basis of mammography, three (15%) required wider excisions on the basis of the sonographic findings. In these three cases, additional foci were demonstrated on ultrasound at distances of 1 cm, 1 cm, and 1.3 cm from the index lesion.

Moon and colleagues [34] performed bilateral breast sonography on 201 patients who had newly diagnosed breast cancer or who were suspected of having breast cancer. In the ipsilateral breasts, sonography depicted 194 (97%) of 201 foci of invasive cancer and 52 (75%) of 69 foci of DCIS. Mammography and physical examination identified 173 (86%) foci of invasive cancer and 56 (81%) foci of DCIS. In the contralateral breasts, ultrasound depicted 11 (92%) of 12 foci of invasive cancer and four (57%) of seven foci of DCIS, whereas mammography and physical examination identified six (50%) foci of invasive cancer and five (71%) foci of DCIS. Sonography identified mammographically and clinically unsuspected multifocal or multicentric cancers in 28 patients (14%) and contralateral cancers in eight patients (4%). On the basis of the sonographic findings, therapy was appropriately changed in 32 patients (16%). In 16 of 18 patients who had multicentric lesions seen on sonography alone, mastectomy was performed instead of lumpectomy. The remaining two patients underwent mastectomy as well because the primary tumors were greater than 3 cm in size.

In the study by Moon and colleagues [34], there were 36 malignant foci in 36 patients detected only on ultrasound, including 24 foci of IDC, four foci of ILC, and eight foci of DCIS. Of these 36 foci, 28 were in the ipsilateral breasts, including 20 foci of IDC, two foci of ILC, and six foci of DCIS. Eight foci were demonstrated in the contralateral breasts, including four foci of IDC, two foci of ILC, and two foci of DCIS [34].

Moon and colleagues [34] noted that patients who have large palpable tumors and those who have dense mammary parenchyma are most likely to have additional tumors detected with bilateral whole breast ultrasound. Of the 36 additional tumors found on ultrasound, 78% were found in patients who had an index tumor greater than 2 cm in size, and 22% were found in patients who had index cancers measuring 2 cm or less. Ninety-two percent of the additional cancers detected with sonography were in mammographically dense breast parenchyma, and 8% of the additional tumors were in fatty breasts. Moon and colleagues noted that a family history of breast cancer, younger age, and lobular histology were risk factors for bilateral breast cancer.

Axillary lymph node metastases

In 21% of the cases in the series of ILCs analyzed by Selinko and colleagues [13], mulifocality/multicentricity was identified by sonography and proven by ultrasound-guided fine-needle aspiration (FNA). Selinko and colleagues also evaluated the axillary, infraclavicular, supraclavicular, and internal mammary lymph node basins with ultrasound. Lymph nodes were considered abnormal if there was evidence of cortical thickening or lobulation, hilar compression, or disappearance of the hilar fat.

In the study by Selinko and colleagues [13], ultrasound-guided FNA (Fig. 12) confirmed evidence of metastatic disease in the axillary lymph nodes in 21% of the cases. Ultrasound-guided axillary lymph node FNA was performed in 18 (29%) of the 62 patients. Eight (44%) of these 18 patients had no palpable lymphadenopathy on clinical examination, and FNA revealed metastatic axillary lymphadenopathy in six patients. In the other two patients, the results of ultrasound-guided axillary FNA were negative; and in one of those cases, axillary lymph node dissection demonstrated a single 2-mm micrometastasis. Ten patients presented with palpable axillary lymphadenopathy. In 3 of these 10 patients, axillary lymph node FNA showed no evidence of metastatic disease. One FNA was false negative due to sampling error, and axillary lymph node dissection revealed that 3 of 17 lymph nodes were positive for ILC. In 7 of the 10 patients who had palpable axillary lymphadenopathy, axillary lymph node FNA confirmed the presence of metastatic disease.

Selinko and colleagues [13] noted that patients who have biopsy-proven axillary metastatic disease are directed to axillary lymph node dissection rather than sentinel lymph node biopsy. In addition, at The University of Texas M. D. Anderson Cancer Center, patients who have known metastatic axillary lymphadenopathy are referred for neoadjuvant chemotherapy before surgery. Patients who have negative axillary lymph node biopsies and small (<2 cm) breast tumors are directed to sentinel lymph node biopsy and surgical excision. In patients who have ILCs greater than 2 cm in greatest dimension, neoadjuvant chemotherapy is administered before surgical excision.

Combined mammography, sonography, and MR imaging

Kneeshaw and colleagues [35] analyzed the findings on mammography, sonography, and MR imaging in 21 women who had ILC. The authors noted that MR imaging detected all 11 cases of subsequently proven multifocal disease, with a positive predictive value of 100% and a negative predictive value of 95%. Mammography and sonography combined identified 3 of the 11 cases (27%) of multifocal disease, with a positive predictive value of 100% and a negative predictive value of 56%. In 5 of 21 cases (24%), clinical management was changed on the basis of the MR imaging findings. The authors concluded that MR imaging should be used for preoperative staging in patients who have ILC.

Berg and colleagues [36] performed bilateral mammography, sonography, and MR imaging in 111 consecutive women who had known or suspected invasive breast cancer. In nonfatty breasts, sonography and MR imaging were more sensitive for invasive cancer, but MR imaging and sonography could lead to overestimation of the extent of disease. Twenty-nine foci of ILC were evaluated, of which eight (28%) were palpable. Mammography was less sensitive for ILC compared with IDC. Also, mammography was less sensitive for ILC than sonography and MR imaging, with no statistically significant difference in sensitivity between ultrasound and MR imaging. Mammography identified 10 of 29 foci of ILC, sonography depicted 25, and MR imaging identified 28. Two foci of ILC were identified only on MR imaging, and one focus of ILC was identified only on second-look ultrasound. Mammography and sonography, with or without clinical examination, identified 25 of 29 (86%) foci of ILC. Mammography, clinical examination, and MR imaging identified 28 of 29 (96%) of foci. Adding sonography or MR imaging to mammography and clinical examination significantly improved the detection of ILC. Mammographic sensitivity for ILC was inversely related to mammographic breast density. Breast density did not affect the sensitivity of MR imaging or ultrasound.

In the study by Berg and colleagues [36], breast conservation therapy was anticipated in 12 breasts with ILC. Sonography and MR imaging (Fig. 13) accurately depicted the extent of disease in eight and seven of those breasts, respectively, compared with five for mammography. In two breasts, mammographically and clinically unsuspected contralateral ILC was identified on the basis of findings on sonography and MR imaging. Berg and colleagues noted that it may be difficult to distinguish ILC from LCIS on sonography and MR imaging.

Summary

In patients who have known or suspected ILC, sonography has been commonly performed after mammography. Now, as more preoperative MR imaging studies are being done, sonography is often performed after MR imaging. Whether ultrasound is done after mammography, after MR imaging, or after both studies, it is important that the person performing the ultrasound study carefully review all prior imaging studies. Although meticulous attention should be paid to the region of the mammographic or the MR imaging abnormality, the remainder of the breast and the contralateral breast should be studied in a careful manner because ILC foci may be occult on mammography or MR imaging but detectable on sonography. Ultrasound along with sonographically guided biopsy can be undertaken to document the presence of ILC; to determine the extent of disease, including the presence of multifocal, multicentric, and contralateral disease; and to stage the regional lymph node basins. Sonography is an invaluable tool in the diagnosis, triage, and management of patients who have ILC.

Acknowledgments

We thank Barbara Almarez Mahinda for assistance in manuscript preparation.

References

[1] Krecke KN, Gisvold JJ. Invasive lobular carcinoma of the breast: mammographic findings and extent of disease at diagnosis in 184 patients. AJR Am J Roentgenol 1993;161(5): 957–60.
[2] Arpino G, Bardou VJ, Clark GM, et al. Infiltrating lobular carcinoma of the breast: tumor characteristics and clinical outcome. Breast Cancer Res 2004;6(3):R149–56.
[3] Bouvet M, Ollila DW, Hunt KK, et al. Role of conservation therapy for invasive lobular carcinoma of the breast. Ann Surg Oncol 1997;4(8): 650–4.
[4] Cornford EJ, Wilson AR, Athanassiou E, et al. Mammographic features of invasive lobular and invasive ductal carcinoma of the breast: a comparative analysis. Br J Radiol 1995;68(809): 450–3.
[5] Helvie MA, Paramagul C, Oberman HA, et al. Invasive lobular carcinoma: imaging features and clinical detection. Invest Radiol 1993;28(3): 202–7.
[6] Newstead GM, Baute PB, Toth HK. Invasive lobular and ductal carcinoma: mammographic findings and stage at diagnosis. Radiology 1992; 184(3):623–7.
[7] Dixon JM, Anderson TJ, Page DL, et al. Infiltrating lobular carcinoma of the breast: an evaluation of the incidence and consequence of bilateral disease. Br J Surg 1983;70(9):513–6.
[8] Lesser ML, Rosen PP, Kinne DW. Multicentricity and bilaterality in invasive breast carcinoma. Surgery 1982;91(2):234–40.
[9] Cocquyt V, Van Belle S. Lobular carcinoma in situ and invasive lobular cancer of the breast. Curr Opin Obstet Gynecol 2005;17(1):55–60.
[10] Cristofanilli M, Gonzalez-Angulo A, Sneige N, et al. Invasive lobular carcinoma classic type: response to primary chemotherapy and survival outcomes. J Clin Oncol 2005;23(1):41–8.
[11] Hilleren DJ, Andersson IT, Lindholm K, et al. Invasive lobular carcinoma: mammographic findings in a 10-year experience. Radiology 1991; 178(1):149–54.
[12] Rosen PP. Invasive lobular carcinoma. In: Rosen PP, editor. Rosen's breast pathology. 2nd edition. Philadelphia: Lipincott Williams & Wilkins; 2001. p. 627–52.
[13] Selinko VL, Middleton LP, Dempsey PJ. Role of sonography in diagnosing and staging invasive lobular carcinoma. J Clin Ultrasound 2004; 32(7):323–32.
[14] Dixon JM, Anderson TJ, Page DL, et al. Infiltrating lobular carcinoma of the breast. Histopathology 1982;6(2):149–61.
[15] Le Gal M, Ollivier L, Asselain B, et al. Mammographic features of 455 invasive lobular carcinomas. Radiology 1992;185(3):705–8.
[16] Harvey JA, Fechner RE, Moore MM. Apparent ipsilateral decrease in breast size at mammography: a sign of infiltrating lobular carcinoma. Radiology 2000;214(3):883–9.
[17] Evans WP, Warren Burhenne LJ, Laurie L, et al. Invasive lobular carcinoma of the breast: mammographic characteristics and computer-aided detection. Radiology 2002;225(1):182–9.
[18] Skaane P, Skjorten F. Ultrasonographic evaluation of invasive lobular carcinoma. Acta Radiol 1999;40(4):369–75.
[19] Bartella L, Liberman L, Morris EA, et al. Nonpalpable mammographically occult invasive breast cancers detected by MRI. AJR Am J Roentgenol 2006;186(3):865–70.
[20] Weinstein SP, Orel SG, Heller R, et al. MR imaging of the breast in patients with invasive lobular carcinoma. AJR Am J Roentgenol 2001;176(2): 399–406.
[21] Yeh ED, Slanetz PJ, Edmister WB, et al. Invasive lobular carcinoma: spectrum of enhancement and morphology on magnetic resonance imaging. Breast J 2003;9(1):13–8.
[22] Chapellier C, Balu-Maestro C, Bleuse A, et al. Ultrasonography of invasive lobular carcinoma of the breast sonographic patterns and diagnostic value report of 102 cases. Clin Imaging 2000; 24(6):333–6.
[23] Cawson JN, Law E-M, Kavanagh AM. Invasive lobular carcinoma: sonographic features of cancers detected in a BreastScreen Program. Australas Radiol 2001;45(1):25–30.
[24] Watermann DO, Tempfer C, Hefler LA, et al. Ultrasound morphology of invasive lobular breast cancer is different compared with other types of breast cancer. Ultrasound Med Biol 2005;31(2):167–74.
[25] Ohta T, Tsujimoto F, Nakajima Y, et al. Ultrasonographic findings of invasive lobular carcinoma differentiation of invasive lobular carcinoma from invasive ductal carcinoma by ultrasonography. Breast Cancer 2005;12(4):304–11.

[26] Rissanen T, Tikkakoski T, Autio AL, et al. Ultrasonography of invasive lobular breast carcinoma. Acta Radiol 1998;39(3):285–91.

[27] Butler RS, Venta LA, Wiley EL, et al. Sonographic evaluation of infiltrating lobular carcinoma. AJR Am J Roentgenol 1999;172(2):325–30.

[28] Ashkar L, Phancao J-P, Mesurolle B. Atypical sonographic appearance of small invasive lobular carcinoma of the breast. J Clin Ultrasound 2006; 34(2):82–3.

[29] Evans N, Lyons K. The use of ultrasound in the diagnosis of invasive lobular carcinoma of the breast less than 10 mm in size. Clin Radiol 2000;55(4):261–3.

[30] Pritt B, Ashikaga T, Oppenheimer RG, et al. Influence of breast cancer histology on the relationship between ultrasound and pathology tumor size measurements. Mod Pathol 2004;17(8):905–10.

[31] Moore MM, Borossa G, Imbrie JZ, et al. Association of infiltrating lobular carcinoma with positive surgical margins after breast-conservation therapy. Ann Surg 2000;231(6):877–82.

[32] Wilkinson LS, Given-Wilson R, Hall T, et al. Increasing the diagnosis of multifocal primary breast cancer by the use of bilateral whole-breast ultrasound. Clin Radiol 2005;60(5):573–8.

[33] Berg WA, Gilbreath PL. Multicentric and multifocal cancer: whole-breast US in preoperative evaluation. Radiology 2000;214(1):59–66.

[34] Moon WK, Noh D-Y, Im J-G. Multifocal, multicentric, and contralateral breast cancers: bilateral whole-breast US in the preoperative evaluation of patients. Radiology 2002;224(2): 569–76.

[35] Kneeshaw PJ, Turnbull LW, Smith A, et al. Dynamic contrast enhanced magnetic resonance imaging aids the surgical management of invasive lobular breast cancer. Eur J Surg Oncol 2003;29(1):32–7.

[36] Berg WA, Gutierrez L, NessAiver MS, et al. Diagnostic accuracy of mammography, clinical examination, US, and MR imaging in preoperative assessment of breast cancer. Radiology 2004;233(3):830–49.

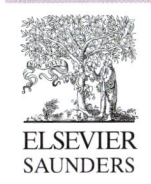

Sonography of Unusual Breast Neoplasms

Wei Tse Yang, MBBS, FRCR*

- Malignant nonepithelial tumors
  Primary lymphoreticular malignancies
  Secondary lymphoreticular malignancies
  Hematogenous metastases
  Sarcomas
  Carcinosarcomas
- Benign tumors

Granular cell tumor
Fibromatosis
- Systemic diseases
  Collagen vascular diseases
  Diabetic fibrous mastopathy
- Summary
- References

Nonepithelial malignancies of the breast are an important minority of breast neoplasms, including primary and metastatic lymphoreticular malignancies, hematogenous metastases from nonmammary malignancies, primary breast sarcomas, and treatment-related breast sarcomas. Rare benign breast tumors and some systemic conditions can mimic primary breast carcinoma clinically and on imaging studies. With increased detection of breast lesions, these nonepithelial and rare benign breast tumors have become more critical in the differential diagnosis of benign- and indeterminate-appearing lesions. Each tumor type has a distinct clinical profile, including presentation, available therapeutic options, and prognosis, underscoring the importance of timely recognition. It is important for radiologists to be familiar with the mammographic, sonographic, and MR imaging appearances of a variety of unusual breast neoplasms because these lesions present diagnostic challenges. Specifically, solitary metastases and uncommon benign lesions must be distinguished from primary epithelial carcinomas of the breast to avoid unnecessary mutilating surgery that does not improve the clinical outcome. This article describes the sonographic features of these uncommon breast neoplasms and systemic conditions.

Malignant nonepithelial tumors

Primary lymphoreticular malignancies

Primary lymphoreticular malignancies are rare. Primary lymphoma of the breast is the most common primary lymphoreticular malignancy, and it accounts for 0.1% to 0.5% of all breast masses. The ratio of primary breast lymphoma to primary breast carcinoma diagnoses is 1:1000 [1,2]. The diagnostic criteria for primary lymphoma of the breast proposed by Wiseman and Liao [1] in 1972 require sufficient material to allow a diagnosis, mammary tissue and lymphomatous infiltrate in close association, the absence of concurrent disseminated disease or prior extramammary lymphoma, and the presence of ipsilateral concurrent axillary nodal involvement. Primary breast lymphoma has been described most frequently in middle-aged and older patients; the incidence of the disease peaks in the sixth decade [2]. Recently, an increasing incidence

---

Department of Diagnostic Radiology, The University of Texas M. D. Anderson Cancer Center, 1515 Holcombe Boulevard, Unit 1350, Houston, TX, 77030, USA
* Correspondence. Department of Diagnostic Radiology, The University of Texas M. D. Anderson Cancer Center, Box 57, 1515 Holcombe Boulevard, Houston, TX 77030-4009.
E-mail address: wyang@di.mdacc.tmc.edu

of primary breast lymphoma in young patients has been reported and also was observed in the author's practice [3]. A higher prevalence of primary breast lymphoma in the right breast than in the left breast has also been reported [2,3].

The mammographic findings associated with primary lymphoma of the breast are nonspecific. For example, in Hodgkin's B-cell lymphoma, mammography may reveal diffuse increased density with associated global skin thickening or a large central lobulated breast mass (Fig. 1) [3–7]. Associated ipsilateral axillary lymphadenopathy is reported in as many as half of the cases [4,6,7]. Sonography may demonstrate diffuse hypoechogenicity within the breast parenchyma that infiltrates the tissues (see Fig. 1), a large heterogeneous hypoechoic solid mass with irregular or indistinct margins, or a markedly hypoechoic mass with a pseudocystic configuration [3]. There frequently is overlying skin and subcutaneous thickening and edema, with occasional dilated lymphatic channels (see Fig. 1). Color Doppler imaging usually reveals hypervascularity. Ipsilateral lymphadenopathy may involve the axillary, infraclavicular, internal mammary, and supraclavicular nodal basins. MR imaging of lymphoma may reveal avidly enhancing focal masses with washout kinetics [3,8].

Primary lymphoreticular malignancies generally respond well to chemotherapy and show early resolution on all imaging abnormalities, with a return of normal morphologic characteristics in the breast on mammography and sonography (see Fig. 1) [3].

Secondary lymphoreticular malignancies

Secondary lymphoreticular malignancies include lymphoma (Fig. 2), leukemia, and myeloma (Fig. 3) [6,7,9,10]. Patients who have secondary lymphoreticular malignancies usually have disseminated disease and a primary tumor that is not located in the breast. Clinically, the patient may have one or more palpable masses. Mammography reveals one or more masses with circumscribed or indistinct margins (see Figs. 2, 3) or focal asymmetric densities [6,7,9,10]. Sonography reveals hypoechoic masses with circumscribed (see Fig. 3) or ill-defined margins [6]. Clinical correlation is vital because differentiating a neoplasm from superimposed infection on the basis of imaging features alone may be difficult in these frequently immunocompromised patients (Fig. 4).

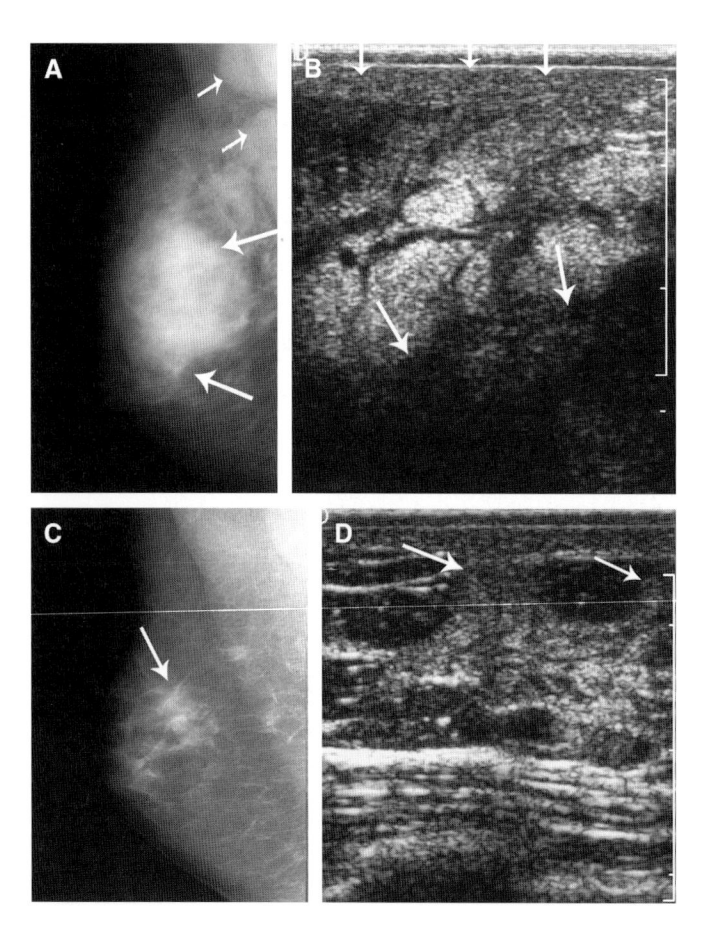

Fig. 1. A 35-year-old woman who has primary non-Hodgkin's B-cell lymphoma of the breast. (*A*) Right mediolateral oblique mammogram shows a large central focal asymmetric density (*long arrow*) with associated ipsilateral axillary lymphadenopathy (*short arrow*). (*B*) Right breast transverse sonogram shows diffuse, abnormal, markedly hypoechoic central echoes (*long arrows*) with overlying skin and subcutaneous edema (*short arrows*). (*C*) Right mediolateral oblique mammogram 4 months after initiation of chemotherapy shows significant resolution of the large central right tumor mass with minimal residual central density (*arrow*). (*D*) Follow-up right breast transverse sonogram shows minimal residual thickening of the overlying Cooper's ligaments (*arrows*) but no significant residual solid mass. (*From* Yang WT, Metreweli C. Sonography of nonmammary malignancies of the breast. AJR Am J Roentgenol 1999;172(2):345; with permission.)

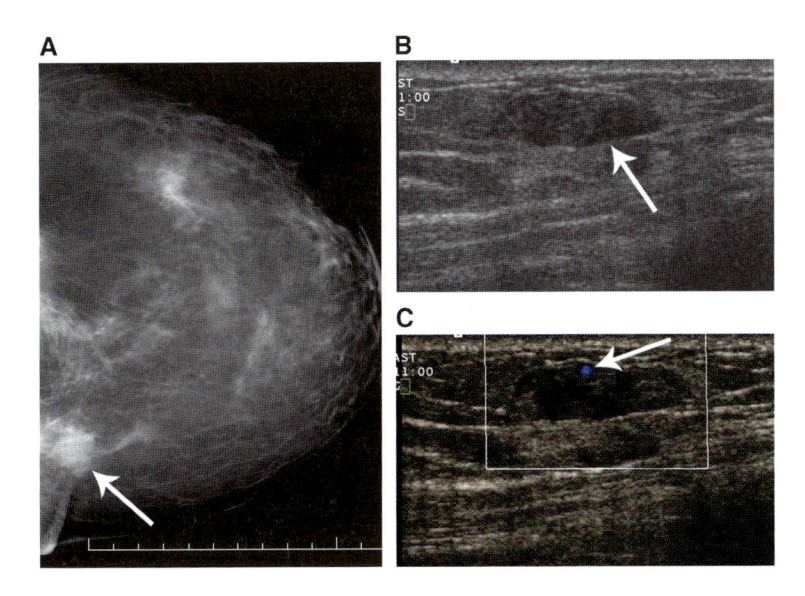

Fig. 2. A 55-year-old woman presented with a new mass in the left breast. The final pathologic examination showed bilateral secondary lymphoma. (*A*) Left craniocaudal mammogram shows a lobular high density mass with indistinct margins (*arrow*) in the upper inner quadrant. (*B*) Left breast transverse sonogram shows a solid, oval, homogeneously hypoechoic mass (*arrow*). (*C*) Color Doppler sonogram of the left breast shows increased peripheral vascularity (*arrow*).

Granulocytic sarcomas are malignant neoplasms of myelogenous origin. One such neoplasm, chloroma, was described by King [11] in 1853 and was named for the green staining caused by myeloperoxidase in the tumor cells. In 1893, Dork [12] described the association between chloroma and leukemia. Granulocytic sarcoma is a solid, invasive, destructive tumor composed of immature cells of the granulocytic series [13]. It is rare in the breast and is more common in bone, lymph nodes, skin,

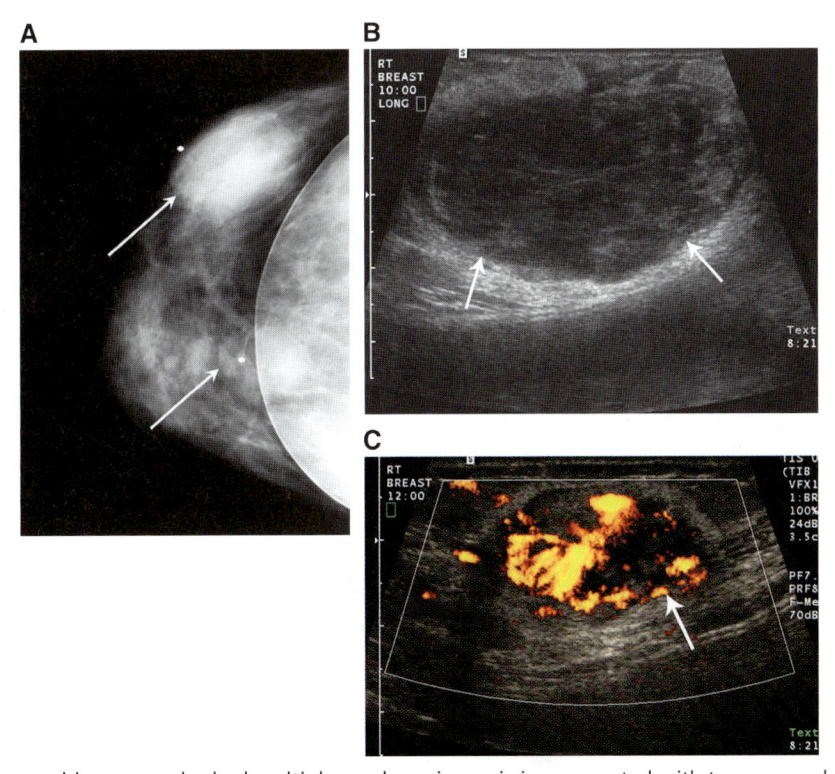

Fig. 3. A 39-year-old woman who had multiple myeloma in remission presented with two new palpable masses in the right breast. (*A*) Right craniocaudal mammogram shows two oval, high-density masses with relatively circumscribed margins (*arrows*) in the right breast, noted by overlying metal markers. (*B*) Transverse sonogram of the right breast at the 9:00 position shows a solid, heterogeneously hypoechoic mass with indistinct boundaries (*arrows*). (*C*) Transverse power Doppler sonogram in the 12:00 position of the right breast position shows a solid hypoechoic oval mass with florid internal hypervascularity (*arrow*).

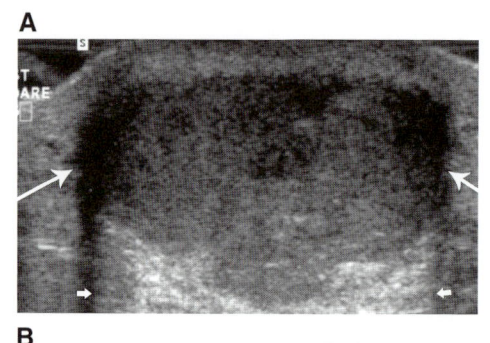

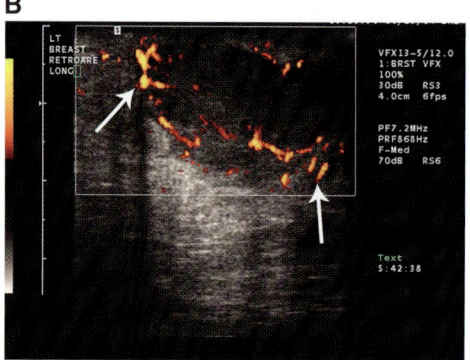

Fig. 4. A 57-year-old man who had acute myelocytic leukemia presented with an acute-onset tender swelling of the left breast during chemotherapy. A fine-needle aspiration yielded polymorphonuclear cells consistent with an abscess. (*A*) Left breast transverse retroareolar sonogram shows a relatively circumscribed, solid hypoechoic mass with indistinct margins (*long arrows*), overlying skin thickening, and posterior acoustic enhancement (*short arrows*). The sonographic features are indistinguishable from a neoplasm; therefore biopsy was necessary. (*B*) Transverse power Doppler sonogram of the left retroareolar lesion shows peripheral hypervascularity (*arrows*).

and soft tissue. Granulocytic sarcoma occurs in association with acute myelogenous leukemia in 3% to 9% of patients [14]. Granulocytic sarcoma is seen often in young women and is frequently bilateral. The mammographic features include one or more circumscribed nodules, and sonography usually reveals hypoechoic nodules [14–16]. Imaging studies do not reliably distinguish granulocytic sarcomas (Fig. 5) from other hematogenous metastases or from primary breast carcinoma.

Hematogenous metastases

Metastases to the breast occur infrequently. The most common metastatic lesions are from primary melanomas (Fig. 6), lung, ovarian, and thyroid carcinomas and soft tissue sarcomas [7,9,17–19]. Metastases to the breast in men are infrequent and occur mainly in patients who have malignant melanoma and prostatic carcinoma [9,20]. In rare cases, metastases involving the breast may be the presenting feature of malignancy [17,18]. Hematogenous metastases in the breast most commonly consist of one or more discrete nodules that tend to be the same size on palpation and mammography [19]. Clinically, breast metastases are palpable, round masses that are firm and freely mobile, without fixation to the skin or the underlying pectoralis muscle. Because these lesions grow rapidly, an important clue to their nature may be a rapid increase in nodule size since the prior mammogram or the prior sonogram [6,7]. Mammography typically reveals circumscribed, round nodules with slightly irregular or indistinct margins (see Fig. 6) [3,6,7,17–19]. There typically is no evidence of spiculation or microcalcifications. Calcifications, when present, tend to represent psammomatous calcifications from ovarian carcinomas [3,9]. The absence of a desmoplastic reaction commonly associated with primary breast epithelial carcinomas may be useful for distinguishing metastases from primary breast carcinomas. Sonography reveals nodules with circumscribed, indistinct, or irregular margins. The lesions may demonstrate echogenic rims (see Fig. 6), and diffuse nodular infiltration of the breast may be present. Color Doppler imaging has revealed hypervascularity in these lesions [3,6].

Sarcomas

Sarcomas are malignancies of mesenchymal tissue that do not contain an epithelial component. Sarcomas rarely occur as primary breast tumors and account for approximately 0.7% of all breast malignancies [21,22]. The most common breast sarcomas are angiosarcomas, fibrosarcomas, rhabdomyosarcomas, and undifferentiated high-grade sarcomas [23–26]. The incidence of postradiation sarcomas has increased with the increasing use of breast-conserving surgery (Fig. 7) [27,28].

Angiosarcoma of the breast is a rare malignant tumor that generally is considered to have a poor prognosis. Mammary angiosarcoma is a morphologically heterogeneous disease: the histologic grades can be high, intermediate, or low [23,29,30]. Morphologic characteristics, tumor size, and symptom duration are helpful in predicting clinical behavior and prognosis [29,30]. Diagnosing mammary angiosarcoma is difficult because findings on mammography, sonography, cytologic examination, and even limited small biopsies may be negative or nonspecific [23]. Clinical examination is important and should give clues to the diagnosis by the presence of thickening and bluish or purplish discoloration of the skin. A study of 21 cases of primary angiosarcoma of the breast

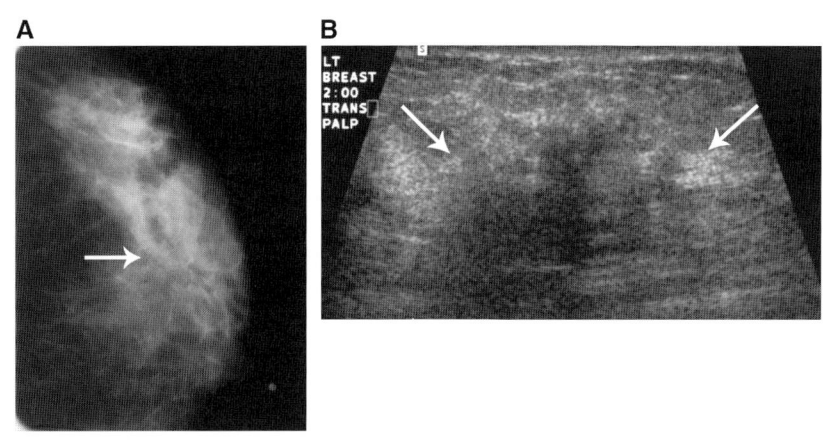

Fig. 5. A 46-year-old woman presented with an acute-onset, palpable, left breast mass while receiving chemotherapy for acute myeloid leukemia. Core needle biopsy was performed, and granulocytic sarcoma was found on histologic examination. (*A*) Left craniocaudal mammogram shows an area of architectural distortion in the upper outer quadrant (*arrow*). (*B*) Transverse left breast sonogram shows an area of architectural distortion (*arrows*).

showed that as many as 33% of the cases were negative on mammography, and up to one third of the cases demonstrated noncalcified masses [23]. Sonography was performed in five cases and revealed echogenic masses [23]. MR imaging also has been used recently, revealing angiosarcoma to have low signal intensity on T1-weighted imaging, high signal intensity on T2-weighted imaging, and several large vessels extending into the lesion, with associated venous lakes [31].

Carcinosarcomas

Carcinosarcomas are the rarest primary malignancies of the breast, accounting for less than 0.1% of cases. The term "carcinosarcoma" originally was proposed by Azzopardi [32] to refer to carcinoma and sarcoma arising together in fibroepithelial lesions of the breast. Subsequently, Wargotz and colleagues [33–36] used the term "metaplastic carcinoma" for tumors with a combination of overt carcinomatous elements and high-grade mesenchymal-appearing areas. These lesions are malignant tumors containing both carcinomatous and sarcomatous components that are derived from both epithelial and mesenchymal elements.

Carcinosarcomas are usually seen in women older than 50 years [33,35,37]. The presenting symptom usually is a palpable mass. The mean tumor size at presentation is 3.3 cm. Some studies have found the tumor size to be the most important

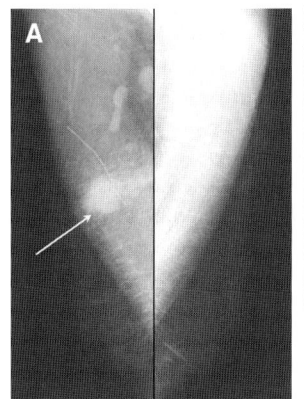

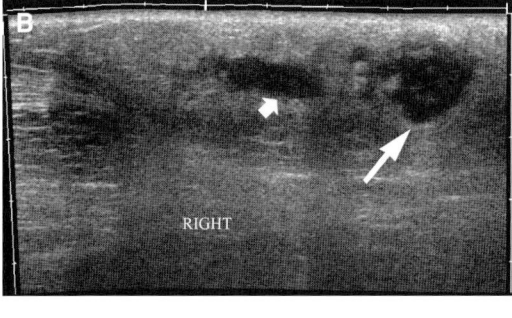

Fig. 6. A 63-year-old man who had malignant melanoma of the left cheek presented with a palpable right axillary tail mass. Pathologic examination showed metastatic melanoma. (*A*) Bilateral mediolateral oblique mammograms show a high-density, oval mass in the right axillary tail, with indistinct margins (*arrow*). (*B*) Extended field of view right axillary tail sonogram shows an irregular hypoechoic mass with indistinct margins (*long arrow*) and tubular ductal extension (*short arrow*). The surrounding margins are indistinct.

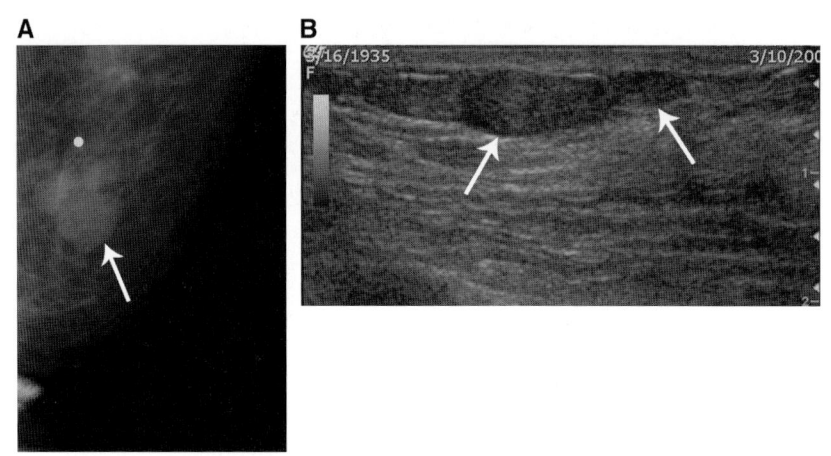

Fig. 7. A 60-year-old woman presented with a palpable mass in the medial left breast 5 years after breast-conserving surgery and radiation therapy. Pathologic examination showed intermediate-grade radiation-associated angiosarcoma. (*A*) Left craniocaudal mammogram shows a lobular, isodense mass with circumscribed margins (*arrow*). The overlying metal marker indicates a palpable finding. (*B*) Left breast transverse sonogram shows a lobular, hypoechoic mass with circumscribed margins (*arrows*).

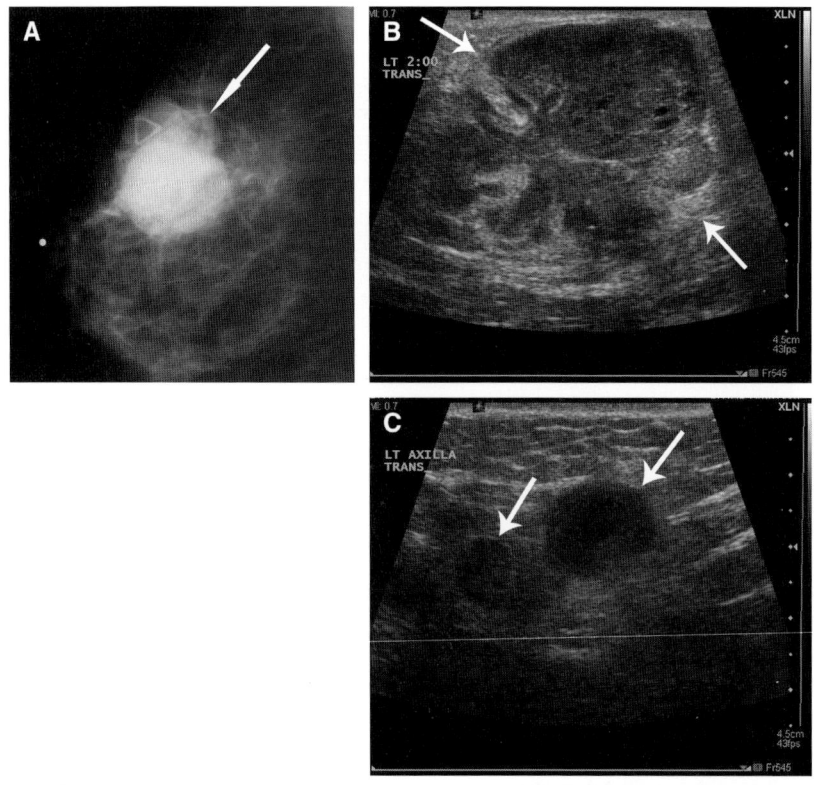

Fig. 8. A 26-year-old woman presented with a rapidly enlarging left breast mass after minor trauma to the breast. Pathologic examination revealed carcinosarcoma. (*A*) Left mediolateral oblique mammogram shows a large, lobular, high-density mass (*arrow*). The overlying triangular marker indicates a palpable finding. (*B*) Left breast transverse sonogram shows a lobular, heterogeneously hypoechoic solid mass (*arrows*). (*C*) Left axillary transverse sonogram shows two abnormal hypoechoic right axillary lymph nodes (*arrows*), representing metastatic disease determined by fine-needle aspiration.

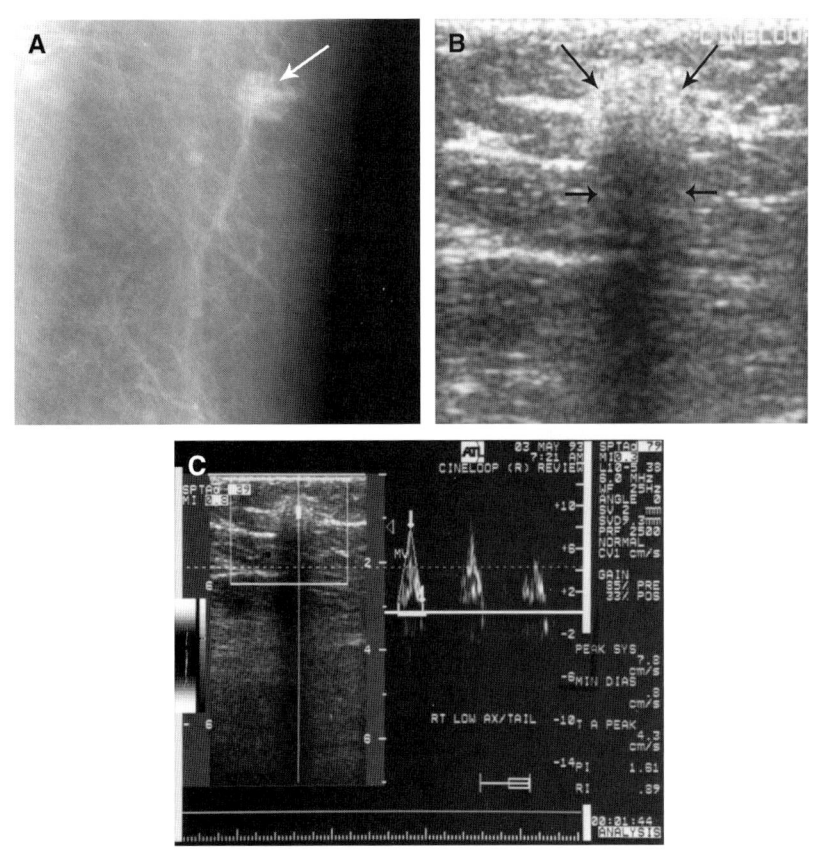

Fig. 9. A 29-year-old woman presented with a palpable left axillary tail mass. Pathologic examination showed a granular cell tumor. (A) Left axillary tail mammogram shows a high-density, round mass with indistinct margins (arrow). (B) Left breast transverse sonogram shows a round, heterogeneously hyperechoic mass (long arrows) with circumscribed margins and marked posterior acoustic shadowing (short arrows). (C) Spectral Doppler imaging shows arterial hypervascularity within the left breast mass.

determinant of patient outcome, and tumors larger than 5 cm are associated with the worst prognosis [36].

Carcinosarcomas have been described as oval, noncalcified masses with circumscribed, indistinct, or obscured margins (Fig. 8), with occasional spicules [38–42]. Carcinosarcomas should be included in the differential diagnosis of predominantly circumscribed, noncalcified masses seen on mammograms. Other tumors that may have similar mammographic features include the triad of circumscribed carcinomas (medullary, papillary, and mucinous carcinomas), phyllodes tumors, and high-grade invasive ductal carcinomas in women who have genetic mutations.

Carcinosarcomas are most frequently seen on sonograms as solid, hypoechoic, hypervascular, oval masses with indistinct margins and posterior acoustic enhancement. Less frequently, carcinosarcomas are seen as microlobulated masses with partially circumscribed margins. Carcinosarcomas with mixed solid and cystic compositions were noted in studies by Park and colleagues [42] and Samuels and colleagues [40], who reported that 5 of 11 (45%) and two of four patients (50%) who had metaplastic carcinomas had mixed solid and cystic tumors, respectively, on sonography.

Benign tumors

Granular cell tumor

Granular cell tumor was first described as a separate clinicopathologic entity in 1926 by Abrikossoff [43] and originally was called "granular cell myoblastoma." Although the lesion originally was thought to arise from muscle, it now is thought to derive from Schwann cells [44]. Approximately 8% of granular cell tumors occur in the breast, usually manifesting as painless, firm, mobile masses in the upper breast. Occasionally, the mass is fixed to the pectoral fascia, the chest wall, or the skin, causing dimpling, retraction, or edema, and simulating breast cancer [45].

The appearance of granular cell tumors on mammographic imaging varies, ranging from a round, circumscribed mass with well-defined margins to an indistinct or a spiculated mass that is indistinguishable from cancer (Fig. 9) [46–49]. Granular cell tumors can appear as new lesions or masses that enlarge over time. Calcifications have not been reported in granular cell tumors. Sonography reveals solid, poorly marginated masses with marked posterior acoustic shadowing or more benign-appearing circumscribed masses [47–49]. Pathologically, granular cell tumors have closely packed nests of cells with abundant cytoplasm containing numerous fine eosinophilic granules [50]. These tumors tend to form syncytial cords and sheets that infiltrate the surrounding tissue and imitate the infiltrative pattern of breast cancer [51,52].

Granular cell tumors in the breast with poorly circumscribed contours may mimic breast cancer. Despite their clinical, mammographic, and sonographic features, which may strongly suggest malignancy, most granular cell tumors are benign, and very few malignant cases have been reported [45,51,52]. Because granular cell tumors of the breast do not show a propensity for aggressive behavior, wide local excision is the treatment of choice.

There have been anecdotal reports of MR imaging and PET studies of granular cell tumors of the breast [53,54]. Kohashi and colleagues [53] described granular cell tumors of the breast as homogeneously enhancing masses on T1-weighted MR imaging, with a rim of high signal intensity on T2-weighted imaging. Hoess and colleagues [54] reported that granular cell tumors of the breast did not show evidence of focally enhanced tracer accumulation on [^{18}F]fluorodeoxyglucose PET. Quantitative image analysis showed a mean standardized uptake value of 1.8, which is below the mean of 2.5 that generally is used to differentiate benign and malignant lesions in the breast.

Fibromatosis

Fibromatosis, also known as extra-abdominal desmoid tumor, is a benign, localized, infiltrating mass composed of fibroblasts and collagen that typically is found in the abdominal wall and rarely is found in the breast. Clinically, there is a single palpable, firm-to-hard nontender mass that is sometimes fixed to the pectoralis fascia. Skin retraction may also be present. The lesion tends to recur locally if not adequately excised, but it has not been found to metastasize [55]. Mammography reveals an irregularly shaped, high-density spiculated mass (Fig. 10) without associated calcifications that is indistinguishable from breast cancer

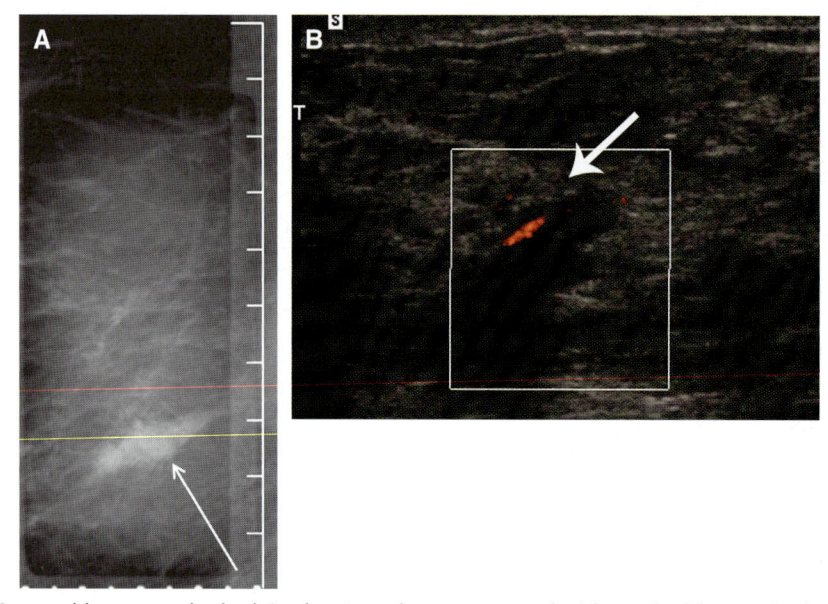

Fig. 10. A 56-year-old woman who had Gardner's syndrome presented with a palpable mass in the right breast. Excisional biopsy showed fibromatosis of the breast. (A) Right lateral mammogram during needle localization shows an elongated elliptical mass (arrow) with indistinct margins. (B) Right breast transverse power Doppler sonogram shows an irregular, solid, hypoechoic mass (arrow) with angular margins and internal hypervascularity.

[56–58]. MR imaging has been reported to demonstrate rapid enhancement, suggestive of malignancy [58]. Sonography reveals an irregular hypoechoic mass with posterior acoustic shadowing that simulates malignancy (see Fig. 10) [59]. Histopathologic examination shows mature fibroblasts arranged in interlacing bundles without nuclear atypia or increased mitotic activity.

Systemic diseases

Systemic diseases infrequently involve the breast, and mammographic and sonographic findings in these cases may be striking and unique. Many systemic conditions have characteristic imaging features in the breast; others may pose a diagnostic challenge because they mimic breast cancer.

Collagen vascular diseases

The most frequent mammographic and sonographic finding associated with collagen vascular disease is bilateral symmetrical lymphadenopathy. The lymphadenopathy is most conspicuous in the axillary regions but frequently also involves the lymph nodes of the neck and the inguinal regions. Generalized lymphadenopathy is associated with collagen vascular disorders such as rheumatoid arthritis, systemic lupus erythematosus, scleroderma, and psoriatic arthritis. Faint metallic deposits may be identified in the axillary lymph nodes in patients who have rheumatoid arthritis who have undergone long-term treatment with gold injections. These deposits may mimic calcifications in metastatic axillary nodes. Other causes of bilateral lymphadenopathy include granulomatous diseases (eg, tuberculosis, sarcoidosis [Fig. 11], and histoplasmosis), AIDS, infectious mononucleosis, lymphoma, and leukemia.

Diabetic fibrous mastopathy

Diabetic fibrous mastopathy was first described in 1984 by Soler and Khardori [60]. It is a benign

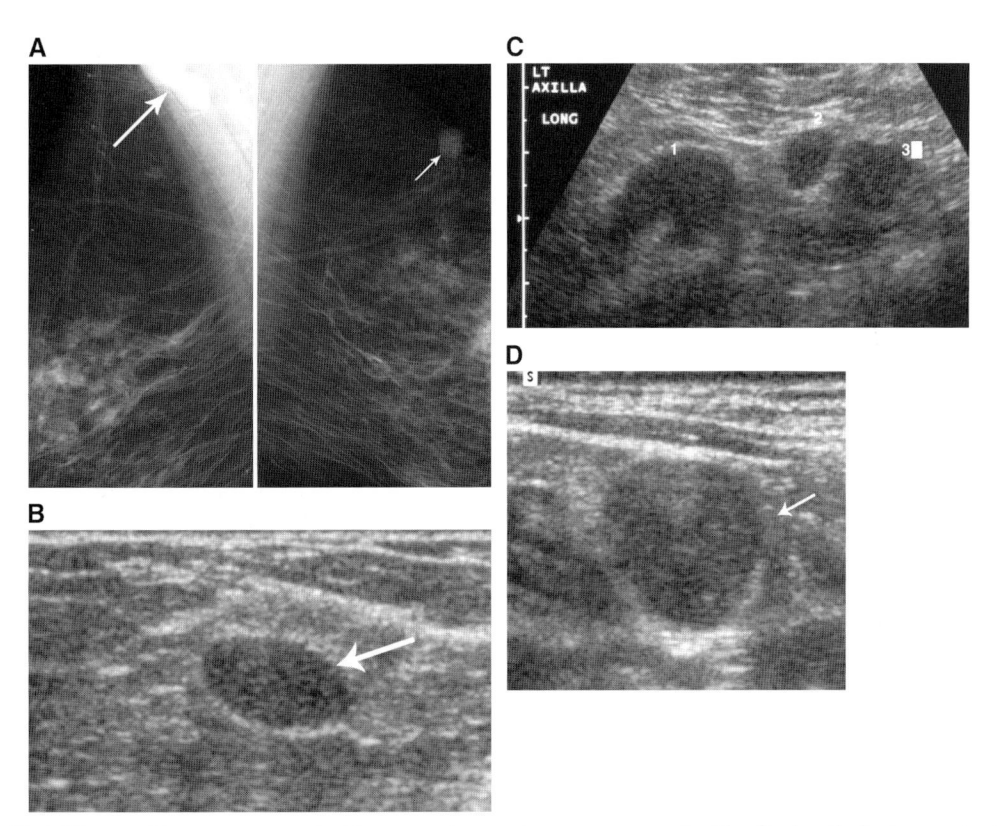

Fig. 11. A 60-year-old woman presented for annual screening mammography. The final pathologic examination of the left intramammary lymph node and the right axillary lymph node showed sarcoidosis. (*A*) Bilateral screening mammograms show an enlarged right axillary lymph node (*long arrow*) and a prominent left intramammary lymph node (*short arrow*). (*B*) Left breast transverse sonogram shows an ovoid, solid, hypoechoic left intramammary lymph node (*arrow*) with loss of the central fatty hilum. (*C*) Left axillary longitudinal sonogram shows enlarged lymph nodes (numbered *1*, *2*, and *3*) with eccentric cortical hypertrophy. (*D*) Left supraclavicular sonogram shows an enlarged, solid, homogeneously hypoechoic lymph node (*arrow*) with loss of the central fatty hilum.

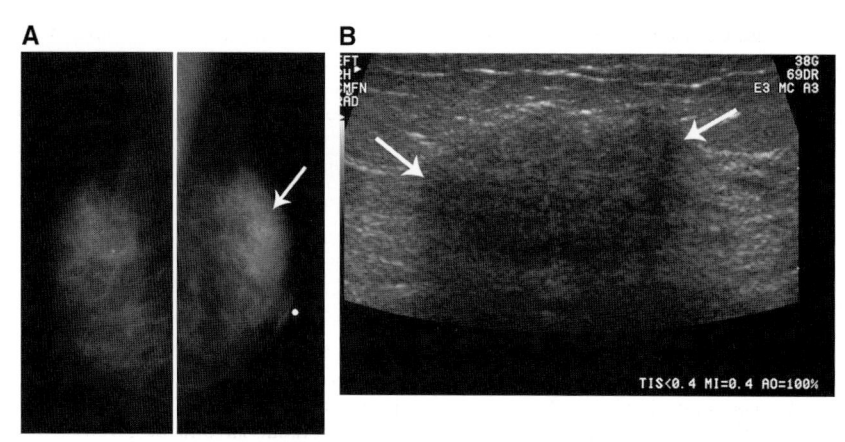

Fig. 12. A 53-year-old woman who had a 5-year history of insulin-dependent diabetes presented with a palpable left breast mass. The final pathologic examination showed B-cell lymphocytic ductitis and lobulitis with varying degrees of keloidal fibrosis, vasculitis, and epithelioid fibroblasts, consistent with diabetic mastopathy. (*A*) Bilateral mediolateral oblique mammograms show a focal asymmetric density in the left upper outer quadrant (*arrow*) with no discrete mass. (*B*) Left breast transverse sonogram shows heterogeneous echoes with posterior acoustic shadowing (*arrows*). No discrete mass was identified on sonography.

condition found In patients who have type 1 insulin-dependent diabetes mellitus and generally manifests with microvascular complications approximately 20 years after the onset of diabetes. Benign fibrous proliferation also has been described in non–insulin-dependent patients [61], patients who have other endocrine diseases, particularly thyroid diseases [60], and, rarely, in men [61]. Up to 60% of diabetic fibrous mastopathy lesions are multicentric, bilateral, or both [60–62]. Recurrent disease, in either the same or the contralateral breast, has been reported [61,62]. Diabetic fibrous mastopathy tends to occur at the same site and to involve more breast tissue than the first lesion, lending support to the theory that surgery may exacerbate the condition.

Diabetic fibrous mastopathy usually presents with a palpable, nontender, hard mass that clinically is indistinguishable from malignancy. On mammography, it has been described as regional and asymmetric, with increased opacity and no discrete mass or spiculation (Fig. 12) [61,63]. On ultrasound, diabetic fibrous mastopathy is characterized by marked posterior acoustic shadowing, with or without an associated ill-defined heterogeneous, hypoechoic mass [61,63]. An atypical presentation with circumscribed nodules has been reported [64]. In addition, color Doppler imaging shows no hypervascularity, which may help in differentiating diabetic fibrous mastopathy, with a relatively avascular histologic profile, from primary breast carcinoma [63].

In the appropriate clinical setting, ultrasound-guided core biopsy currently is considered adequate for diagnosis. Excisional biopsy is recommended only in the presence of additional clinical or imaging features that are highly suggestive of malignancy. Histologically, the presence of lymphocytic (primarily B-cell) ductitis and lobulitis with varying degrees of keloidal fibrosis, vasculitis, and epithelioid fibroblasts [62] should lead to a diagnosis of diabetic fibrous mastopathy.

Summary

The various manifestations of unusual breast neoplasms—ranging from no imaging abnormalities in a young patient with a clinical finding such as a palpable mass, to a benign appearance or overtly malignant imaging features—should be kept in mind. It is important to recognize the varied features of unusual breast neoplasms and systemic conditions affecting the breast because the prognosis and the management algorithms differ significantly for each disease and from those of primary breast carcinoma.

References

[1] Wiseman C, Liao KT. Primary lymphoma of the breast. Cancer 1972;29(6):1705–12.
[2] Petrek JA. Lymphoma. In: Harris JR, Hellman S, Henderson IC, et al, editors. Breast diseases. 2nd edition. Philadelphia: Lippincott; 1991. p. 806–7.
[3] Yang WT, Muttarak M, Ho LWC. Nonmammary malignancies of the breast: ultrasound, CT, and MRI. Semin Ultrasound CT MR 2000;21(5): 375–94.

[4] Liberman L, Giess CS, Dershaw DD, et al. Non-Hodgkin lymphoma of the breast: imaging characteristics and correlation with histopathologic findings. Radiology 1994;192(1):157–60.
[5] Jackson FI, Lalani ZH. Breast lymphoma: radiologic imaging and clinical appearances. Can Assoc Radiol J 1991;42(1):48–54.
[6] Paulus DD. Lymphoma of the breast. Radiol Clin North Am 1990;(4);28:833–40.
[7] Yang WT, Metreweli C. Sonography of nonmammary malignancies of the breast. AJR Am J Roentgenol 1999;172(2):343–8.
[8] Mussurakis S, Carleton PJ, Turnbull LW. MR imaging of primary non-Hodgkin's lymphoma. A case report. Acta Radiol 1997;38(1):104–7.
[9] Paulus DD, Libshitz HI. Metastasis to the breast. Radiol Clin North Am 1982;20(3):561–8.
[10] Feder JM, Shaw de Paredes E, Hogge JP, et al. Unusual breast lesions: radiologic-pathologic correlation. Radiographics 1999;19:S11–26.
[11] King A. A case of chloroma. Monthly Journal of Medicine 1853;17:97.
[12] Dork G. Chloroma and its relation to leukemia. Am J Med Sci 1893;106:152.
[13] Rappaport H. Tumors of hematopoietic system. In: Atlas of tumor pathology, section 3, fascicle 8. Washington, DC: Armed Forces Institute of Pathology; 1966. p. 239–85.
[14] Barloon TJ, Young DC, Bass SH. Multicentric granulocytic sarcoma (chloroma) of the breast: mammographic findings. AJR Am J Roentgenol 1993;161(5):963–4.
[15] Hiorns MP, Murfitt J. Granulocytic sarcoma (chloroma) of the breast: sonographic findings. AJR Am J Roentgenol 1997;169(6):1639–40.
[16] Son HJ, Oh KK. Multicentric granulocytic sarcoma of the breast: mammographic and sonographic findings. AJR Am J Roentgenol 1998;171(1):274–5.
[17] Toombs BD, Kalisher L. Metastatic disease to the breast: clinical, pathologic, and radiographic features. AJR Am J Roentgenol 1977;129(4):673–6.
[18] Amichetti M, Perani B, Boi S. Metastases to the breast from extramammary malignancies. Oncology 1990;47(3):257–60.
[19] Bohman LG, Bassett LW, Gold RH, et al. Breast metastases from extramammary malignancies. Radiology 1982;144(2):309–12.
[20] Salyer WR, Salyer DC. Metastases of prostatic carcinoma to the breast. J Urol 1973;109(4):671–4.
[21] D'Orsi CJ, Feldhaus L, Sonnenfeld M. Unusual lesions of the breast. Radiol Clin North Am 1983;21(1):67–80.
[22] Berg JW, Decosse JJ, Fracchia AA, et al. Stromal sarcomas of the breast. A unified approach to connective tissue sarcomas other than cystosarcoma phyllodes. Cancer 1962;15:418–24.
[23] Liberman L, Dershaw DD, Kaufman RJ, et al. Angiosarcoma of the breast. Radiology 1992;183(3):649–54.
[24] Elson BC, Ikeda DM, Andersson I, et al. Fibrosarcoma of the breast: mammographic findings in five cases. AJR Am J Roentgenol 1992;158(5):993–5.
[25] Yang WT, Kwan WH, Chow LT, et al. Unusual sonographic appearance with color Doppler imaging of bilateral breast metastases in a patient with alveolar rhabdomyosarcoma of an extremity. J Ultrasound Med 1996;15(7):531–3.
[26] Perlet C, Sittek H, Forstpointner R, et al. Metastases to the breast from rhabdomyosarcoma: appearances on MRI. Eur Radiol 1999;9(6):1113–6.
[27] Mark RJ, Poen J, Tran LM, et al. Postirradiation sarcomas: a single-institution study and review of the literature. Cancer 1994;73(10):2653–62.
[28] Kuten A, Sapir D, Cohen Y, et al. Post irradiation soft tissue sarcoma occurring in breast cancer patients: report of seven cases and results of combination chemotherapy. J Surg Oncol 1985;28(3):168–71.
[29] Donnell RM, Rosen PP, Lieberman PH, et al. Angiosarcoma and other vascular tumors of the breast. Am J Surg Pathol 1981;5(7):629–42.
[30] Gulesserian HP, Lawton RL. Angiosarcoma of the breast. Cancer 1969;24(5):1021–6.
[31] Marchant LK, Orel SG, Perez-Jaffe LA, et al. Bilateral angiosarcoma of the breast on MR imaging. AJR Am J Roentgenol 1997;169(4):1009–10.
[32] Azzopardi JG, Ahmed A, Millis RR. Problems in breast pathology. In: Major problems in pathology, vol. 11. Philadelphia: Saunders; 1979.
[33] Wargotz ES, Norris HJ. Metaplastic carcinoma of the breast. I. Matrix-producing carcinoma. Hum Pathol 1989;20(7):628–35.
[34] Wargotz ES, Deos PH, Norris HJ. Metaplastic carcinoma of the breast. II. Spindle cell carcinoma. Hum Pathol 1989;20(8):732–40.
[35] Wargotz ES, Norris HJ. Metaplastic carcinoma of the breast. IV. Squamous cell carcinoma of ductal origin. Cancer 1990;65(2):272–6.
[36] Wargotz ES, Norris HJ. Metaplastic carcinoma of the breast. III. Carcinosarcoma. Cancer 1989;64(7):1490–9.
[37] Oberman HA. Metaplastic carcinoma of the breast. A clinicopathologic study of 29 patients. Am J Surg Pathol 1987;11(12):918–29.
[38] Gunhan-Bilgen I, Memis A, Ustum EE, et al. Metaplastic carcinoma of the breast: clinical, mammographic, and sonographic findings with histopathologic correlation. AJR Am J Roentgenol 2002;178(6):1421–5.
[39] Patterson SK, Tworek JA, Roubidoux MA, et al. Metaplastic carcinoma of the breast: mammographic appearances with pathologic correlation. AJR Am J Roentgenol 1997;169(3):709–12.
[40] Samuels TH, Miller NA, Manchul LA, et al. Squamous cell carcinoma of the breast. Can Assoc Radiol J 1996;47(3):177–82.
[41] Brenner RJ, Turner RR, Schiller V, et al. Metaplastic carcinoma of the breast: report of three cases. Cancer 1998;82(6):1082–7.
[42] Park JM, Han BK, Moon WK, et al. Metaplastic carcinoma of the breast: mammographic and

sonographic findings. J Clin Ultrasound 2000; 28(4):179–86.
[43] Abrikossoff A. Uber myome, ausgehend von der quergestreiften, wilkurlichen Muskulatur. Virchows Arch Pathol Anat 1926;260:215.
[44] Nathrath WB, Remberger K. Immunohistochemical study of granular cell tumours. Demonstration of neurone specific enolase, S100 protein, laminin and alpha-1-antichymotrypsin. Virchows Arch A Pathol Anat Histopathol 1986; 408(4):421–34.
[45] Khansur T, Balducci L, Tavassoli M. Granular cell tumor. Clinical spectrum of the benign and malignant entity. Cancer 1987;60(2):220–2.
[46] Bassett LW, Cove HC. Myoblastoma of the breast. AJR Am J Roentgenol 1979;132(1):122–3.
[47] Scatarige JC, Hsiu JG, de la Torre R, et al. Acoustic shadowing in benign granular cell tumor (myoblastoma) of the breast. J Ultrasound Med 1987;6(9):545–7.
[48] Baum JK, Robins JR, Schnitt S, et al. The ultrasound appearance of granular cell tumor of the breast: a case report. Breast Dis 1994;7:281–5.
[49] Siegel JR, Sanders L, Kalisher L, et al. Unusual sonographic features of granular cell tumor of the breast. J Ultrasound Med 1999;18(12):857–9.
[50] Sirgi KE, Sneige N, Fanning TV, et al. Fine-needle aspirates of granular cell lesions of the breast: report of three cases, with emphasis on differential diagnosis and utility of immunostaining for CD68 (KP1). Diagn Cytopathol 1996;15(5): 403–8.
[51] Adeniran A, Al-Ahmadie H, Mahoney MC, et al. Granular cell tumor of the breast: a series of 17 cases and review of the literature. Breast J 2004; 10(6):528–31.
[52] Uzoaro I, Firfer B, Ray V, et al. Malignant granular cell tumor. Arch Pathol Lab Med 1992; 116(2):206–8.

[53] Kohashi T, Kataoka T, Haruta R, et al. Granular cell tumor of the breast: report of a case. Hiroshima J Med Sci 1999;48(1):31–3.
[54] Hoess C, Freitag K, Kolben M, et al. FDG PET evaluation of granular cell tumor of the breast. J Nucl Med 1998;39(8):1398–401.
[55] Rosen PP, Ernsberger D. Mammary fibromatosis: a benign spindle-cell tumor with significant risk for local recurrence. Cancer 1989;63(7):1363–9.
[56] Cederlund CG, Gustavsson S, Linell F, et al. Fibromatosis of the breast mimicking carcinoma at mammography. Br J Radiol 1984;57(673): 98–101.
[57] Mesurolle B, Ariche-Cohen M, Mignon F, et al. Unusual mammographic and ultrasonographic findings in fibromatosis of the breast. Eur Radiol 2001;11(11):2241–3.
[58] Lopez-Ruiz J, Ruiz M, Echevarria JJ, et al. Mammary fibromatosis mimicking recurrent breast cancer: radiological findings. Eur Radiol 2005; 15(9):2034–6.
[59] Leibman AJ, Kossoff MB. Sonographic features of fibromatosis of the breast. J Ultrasound Med 1991;10(3):43–5.
[60] Soler NG, Khardori R. Fibrous disease of the breast, thyroiditis, and cheiroarthropathy in type 1 diabetes mellitus. Lancet 1984;1(8370): 193–5.
[61] Logan WW, Hoffman NY. Diabetic fibrous breast disease. Radiology 1989;172(3):667–70.
[62] Ely KA, Tse G, Simpson JF, et al. Diabetic mastopathy: a clinicopathologic review. Am J Clin Pathol 2000;113(4):541–5.
[63] Wong KT, Tse GMK, Yang WT. Ultrasound and MR imaging of diabetic mastopathy. Clin Radiol 2002;57(8):730–5.
[64] Dipiro PJ, Meyer JE, Lester SC. An unusual presentation of lymphocytic mastopathy in a diabetic patient. Clin Radiol 1999;54(12):845–6.

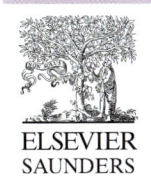

Index

Note: Page numbers of article titles are in **boldface** type.

A

Abscesses, breast, 624–625
Alveolar invasive lobular carcinoma, 646
Angiosarcomas, 664–665
Apocrine ductal carcinoma in situ, 633
Architectural distortion, in mammographic-sonographic correlation, 577–580, 582
Aspiration
    in fine-needle biopsy, 611–612
    of simple breast cysts, 619–622
Asymmetries, in mammographic-sonographic correlation, 577–580
Atypical ductal hyperplasia, versus ductal carcinoma in situ, 632
Axillary metastasis
    from invasive lobular carcinoma, 657–658
    MRI-sonography correlation in, 594–596

B

Benign breast lesions, 667–670. See also Cystic breast lesions.
Bilateral symmetrical lymphadenopathy, 669–670
Bilaterality, of ductal carcinoma in situ, 633
Biopsy, ultrasound-guided, of breast, **603–615**
    advantages of, 603–604
    core-needle, 605–611
    disadvantages of, 604
    fine-needle, 611–612
    in ductal carcinoma in situ, 641
    marker placement in, 612
    pathologic correlation with, 612–613
    preprocedural preparations for, 604–605
    vacuum-assisted, 610–611
    with calcifications, 610
BRCA gene mutations, MRI-sonography correlation in, 594

Breast lesions
    abscesses, 624–625
    benign tumors, 667–670
    biopsy of, **603–615,** 641
    calcifications. See Calcifications.
    carcinosarcomas, 665–667
    cystic. See Cystic breast lesions.
    diabetic fibrous mastopathy, 669–670
    ductal carcinoma in situ. See Ductal carcinoma in situ.
    fibromatosis, 668–669
    genetic predisposition to, 594
    granular cell tumor, 667–668
    in collagen vascular diseases, 669
    in systemic diseases, 669–670
    inflammatory carcinoma, 585–586
    invasive lobular carcinoma, 579, **645–660**
    lymphoreticular malignancies, 661–664
    malignant nonepithelial tumors, 661–664
    mammographic-sonographic correlation of, **567–591**
    metastatic, 646–647, 657–658, 664
    MRI-ultrasonographic correlation of, **593–601**
    nipple discharge from, 587, 625–626
    occult carcinoma, 594–596
    palpable, 587–589
    papillomatous, 625–629, 637
    sarcomas, 663–665
    unusual neoplasms, **661–672**
Breastfeeding, abscess in, 624–625

C

Calcifications
    core biopsy of, 610
    in ductal carcinoma in situ, 635
    in invasive lobular carcinoma, 647–648

Calcifications (*continued*)
    mammographic-sonographic correlation in, 580–584
    simple cysts and, 620
Carcinoma(s)
    inflammatory, mammographic-sonographic correlation in, 585
    intracystic, 619, 622
    invasive lobular. *See* Invasive lobular carcinoma.
    metaplastic (carcinosarcoma), 665–667
    occult, MRI-sonography correlation in, 594–596
    papillary, 629
Carcinoma in situ
    ductal. *See* Ductal carcinoma in situ.
    lobular, 632
Carcinosarcomas, 665–667
Central necrosis, in ductal carcinoma in situ, 632–633
Chloromas, 663–664
Cine clips, in ductal carcinoma in situ, 634
Classic invasive lobular carcinoma, 645–646
Clear cell ductal carcinoma in situ, 633
Clock-face location, in mammography, 568
Clustered microcysts, in ductal carcinoma in situ, 638–640
Collagen vascular diseases, 669–670
Color Doppler imaging, in ductal carcinoma in situ, 634
Complex cystic masses, 629
Core-needle biopsy, ultrasound-guided, 605–611
Craniocaudal mammogram, 568, 570
Cystic breast lesions, 617–625
    abscesses, 624–625
    complex, 629
    galactoceles, 624
    in ductal carcinoma in situ, 637–640
    oil, 622–623
    postoperative, 623–624
    simple, 617–622
    solid mass with, 637
    traumatic, 623–624

D

DCIS. *See* Ductal carcinoma in situ.
Desmoid tumor, 668–669
Diabetic fibrous mastopathy, 669–670
Dilation, of ducts, in ductal carcinoma in situ, 637–638
Doppler imaging, in ductal carcinoma in situ, 634
Ductal carcinoma in situ, **631–643**
    abnormal duct in, 637–638
    anatomy of, 632
    as solid mass, 635–637
    bilaterality of, 633
    calcifications in, 635
    epidemiology of, 631–632
    growth patterns of, 633
    histopathologic prognostic features of, 632–633
    mammographic-sonographic correlation in, 572, 579–582, 584
    mammography in, 633
    margins of, 663
    multicentricity of, 633
    natural history of, 631
    papillary form of, 637
    small cyst clusters in, 638–640
    sonography in
        appearance of, 634–640
        interventional, 640–641
        technique for, 634
    subtypes of, 633
    versus atypical ductal hyperplasia, 632
    versus invasive cancer, 632
    versus lobular carcinoma in situ, 632
Ductal hyperplasia, versus ductal carcinoma in situ, 632
Ducts, abnormalities of, in ductal carcinoma in situ, 637–638

E

Endocrine ductal carcinoma in situ, 633
Epithelial hyperplasia, ductal, versus ductal carcinoma in situ, 632

F

Familial predisposition, to breast cancer, MRI-sonography correlation in, 594
Fat necrosis, oil cyst formation in, 622–623
Fibromatosis, 668–669
Fibrosarcomas, 664
Fibrous mastopathy, diabetic, 669–670
Fine-needle biopsy, ultrasound-guided, 611–612
Fluid collections. *See* Cystic breast lesions.

G

Galactoceles, 624
Galactography, 587
Genetic predisposition, to breast cancer, MRI-sonography correlation in, 594
Granular cell tumor, 667–668
Granulocytic sarcomas, 663–664
Gurgling breast cysts, 617–618

H

Hematogenous metastasis, 664
Hematomas, 624
Hodgkin's disease, 662

I

Implant evaluation, mammographic-sonographic correlation in, 585
Inflammatory carcinoma, mammographic-sonographic correlation in, 585
Interventional sonography, in ductal carcinoma in situ, 640–641
Intracystic carcinomas, 619, 622
Invasive lobular carcinoma, **645–660**
    axillary metastasis from, 657–658
    clinical presentation of, 646–647
    combined imaging in, 658
    epidemiology of, 645
    magnetic resonance imaging in, 648–651, 658
    mammographic-sonographic correlation in, 579, 582
    mammography in, 647–648, 658
    metastasis from, 646–647, 657–658
    multifocal and multicentric, 657
    pathology of, 645–646
    prognosis for, 646
    sonography in, 651–658
    subtypes of, 645–646

L

Landmarks, in mammographic-sonographic correlation, 570, 572
Lateral view, in mammography, 568
Leukemia, 662
Lobular carcinoma in situ, versus ductal carcinoma in situ, 632
Location, in mammographic-sonographic correlation, 567–571
Lumpectomy, cystic fluid collections after, 623–624
Lymphadenopathy, bilateral symmetrical, 669–670
Lymphomas, 661–662
Lymphoreticular malignancies, 661–664

M

Magnetic resonance imaging
    in invasive lobular carcinoma, 648–651, 658
    sonographic correlation with, **593–601**
        clinical decision making in, 599
        in genetic predisposition, 594
        in occult carcinoma, 594–596
        in second-look sonography, 595–597
        pitfalls in, 599–600
        technique for, 598–599
Malignant nonepithelial tumors, 661–665
    carcinosarcomas, 665–667
    hematogenous metastasis, 664
    lymphoreticular, 661–664
    sarcomas, 664–665

Mammographic-sonographic correlation, **567–591**
    architectural distortion in, 577–580, 582
    asymmetries in, 577–580
    challenges in, 577
    confirming concordance in, 589
    in calcifications, 580–584
    in implant evaluation, 585
    in inflammatory carcinoma, 585
    in nipple discharge, 587
    in palpable abnormalities, 587–589
    intrinsic landmarks in, 570, 572
    location in, 567–571
    mass characteristics in, 572–577
    size in, 572
Mammography
    in ductal carcinoma in situ, 633
    in invasive lobular carcinoma, 647–648, 658
    in lymphoma, 662
Margins, of ductal carcinoma in situ, 663
Markers, for biopsy site, 612
Mass characteristics, in mammographic-sonographic correlation, 572–577
Mastitis, abscess in, 624–625
Mastopathy, diabetic fibrous, 669–670
Mediolateral oblique mammogram, 567–568, 570
Metaplastic carcinoma (carcinosarcoma), 665–667
Metastasis
    from invasive lobular carcinoma, 646–647, 657–658
    hematogenous, 664
    MRI-sonography correlation in, 594–596
Microcysts, in ductal carcinoma in situ, 638–640
Mixed type invasive lobular carcinoma, 646
MRI. *See* Magnetic resonance imaging.
Multicentricity
    in ductal carcinoma in situ, 633
    in invasive lobular carcinoma, 657
Multifocal invasive lobular carcinoma, 657
Multiple peripheral papillomas, 627–629
Myeloma, 662

N

Necrosis
    fat, oil cyst formation in, 622–623
    in ductal carcinoma in situ, 632–633
Nipple
    abscess of, 624–625
    as landmark, 570
    discharge from, 587, 625–626
    lesions behind, 568–569, 571
Nonepithelial tumors, malignant, 661–665
Nuclear grade, in ductal carcinoma in situ, 632

O

Occult carcinoma, MRI-sonography correlation in, 594–596
Oil cysts, 622–623

P

Palpable abnormalities, mammographic-sonographic correlation in, 587–589
Papillary carcinoma, 629
Papilloma(s)
    in ductal carcinoma in situ, 637
        multiple peripheral, 627–629
        solitary, 625–627
Peripheral papillomas, 627–629
Pleomorphic invasive lobular carcinoma, 646
Postoperative cystic breast lesions, 623–624
Power Doppler imaging, in ductal carcinoma in situ, 634

Q

Quadrants, in mammography, 567

R

Radiation therapy
    cystic fluid collections after, 623–624
    sarcomas due to, 664
Rhabdomyosarcomas, 664
Rheumatoid arthritis, breast lesions in, 669

S

Sarcomas, 663–665
Scar, as landmark, 570
Signet-ring ductal carcinoma in situ, 633
Simple breast cysts, 617–622
Size, in mammographic-sonographic correlation, 572
Solid invasive lobular carcinoma, 646
Solid mass structure, in ductal carcinoma in situ, 635–637
Solitary papilloma, 625–627
Spiculated mass, in invasive lobular carcinoma, 648
Subareolar abscess, 624–625
Surgery, cystic fluid collections after, 623–624

T

Terminal ductal-lobular units, 632
Trabecular invasive lobular carcinoma, 646
Traumatic cystic breast lesions, 623–624
Triangulation, in mammography, 567–568
Tumors of other histologic differentiation, invasive lobular carcinoma as, 652

V

Vacuum-assisted core biopsy, 610–611

Z

Zuska's disease, 625